Advanced Cardiac
Life Support

ADVANCED CARDIAC LIFE SUPPORT

The practical approach

SECOND EDITION

The Advanced Life Support Group

Edited by

Peter Driscoll
Carl Gwinnutt
Kevin Mackway-Jones
Terry Wardle

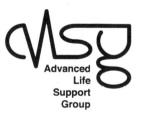

CHAPMAN & HALL MEDICAL
London · Weinheim · New York · Tokyo · Melbourne · Madras

Published by Chapman & Hall, 2–6 Boundary Row, London SE1 8HN, UK

Chapman & Hall, 2–6 Boundary Row, London SE1 8HN, UK

Chapman & Hall GmbH, Pappelallee 3, 69469 Weinheim, Germany

Chapman & Hall USA, 115 Fifth Avenue, New York, NY 10003, USA

Chapman & Hall Japan, ITP-Japan, Kyowa Building, 3F, 2-2-1 Hirakawacho, Chiyoda-ku, Tokyo 102, Japan

Chapman & Hall Australia, 102 Dodds Street, South Melbourne, Victoria 3205, Australia

Chapman & Hall India, R. Seshadri, 32 Second Main Road, CIT East, Madras 600 035, India

First edition 1993
Second edition 1997

© 1993, 1997 Chapman & Hall

Typeset in 12/14pt Palatino by Saxon Graphics Ltd, Derby
Printed in Great Britain by TJ Press International, Padstow, Cornwall

ISBN 0 412 71090 0

A catalogue record for this book is available from the British Library

Library of Congress Catalog Card Number 97-68980

∞ Printed on acid-free text paper, manufactured in accordance with ANSI/NISO Z39.48-1992 and ANSI/NISO Z39.48-1984 (Performanence of Paper).

Contents

Contents

Contents

Contributors

Chris Cahill, FRCS RN
Consultant in Emergency Medicine
Royal Naval Hospital Haslar
Gosport

Patrick Dando, MRCGP
Medical Representative of MDU
Medical Defence Union
London

Peter Driscoll, MD, FRCS
Senior Lecturer in Emergency Medicine
Hope Hospital
Salford

Gill Ellison, SRN
Sister in Emergency Medicine
Hope Hospital
Salford

Carl Gwinnutt, FRCA
Consultant Neuroanaesthetist
Hope Hospital
Salford

Kevin Mackway-Jones, FRCP, FRCS
Consultant in Emergency Medicine
Manchester Royal Infirmary
Manchester

Patrick Nee, MRCP, FRCS
Consultant in Emergency Medicine
Whiston Hospital
Liverpool

Steve Southworth, FRCS
Consultant in Emergency Medicine
Stepping Hill Hospital
Stockport

Terry Wardle, DM, MRCP
Consultant Physician
Countess of Chester Hospital
Chester

Marion Waters, FRCS
Consultant in Emergency Medicine
Countess of Chester Hospital
Chester

Preface

This second edition has been written with the aim of maintaining the objectives of the first edition; namely to enable all healthcare workers to understand the principles of managing a cardiac emergency safely and effectively and to evolve as new procedures and treatments become accepted. Many of the changes have been made to ensure that the reader has an up-to-date description of the UK and European Resuscitation Council guidelines for managing cardiac emergencies. Other changes are in response to the feedback we have received from the many healthcare providers who read the first edition.

The UK is now in the position of having a unified course teaching all aspects of managing cardiac resuscitation, following the amalgamation of the Advanced Life Support Group and Resuscitation Council courses in 1995. We hope that this book will contribute in some way to improving the understanding and management of all patients who have suffered cardiorespiratory distress and will improve their outcome.

We remain convinced that the written word alone cannot teach the practical skills necessary during resuscitation, and readers are encouraged to attend an advanced life support course to obtain these skills.

Ultimately our aims remain unchanged, and as practices and treatments develop this book will continue to change to include them. We are now more certain that it provides a solid and safe foundation of knowledge and skills which can be built upon.

However, it does not represent the end of learning.

Editorial board: Peter Driscoll, Carl Gwinnutt , Kevin Mackway-Jones, Terry Wardle.

Acknowledgements

The Advanced Life Support Group would like to thank, in retro-spect, the Course Directors and their faculties, but mostly the candidates, who, having completed the Advanced Cardiac Life Support Courses, offered constructive criticism which has made this new edition possible.

We are indebted to Mary Harrison MMAA, Keith Harrison AIMBI, MMAA, Denise Smith BA MMAA and Helen Carruthers who successfully translated our descriptions into the line diagrams you see in this book.

The Advanced Life Support Group also gratefully acknowledges the continued support of Laerdal (UK) Ltd, without whose help this course could not have developed to the degree that it has, and for permission to reproduce their artwork for Figures 9.2, 9.3 and 9.4. Sincere thanks are also due to: Hoechst (UK) Ltd for permission to reproduce Figures 8.12, 8.15–8.19, 8.21, 8.22, 8.27 and 9.13 from their excellent ECG Atlas; The British Association for Immediate Care for Figure 14.6 and to Blackwell Science for Figure 14.5 (from *Clinical Anaesthesia*, Carl L Gwinnutt, 1996).

We also wish to thank the ECG Department at Hope Hospital, Salford and the Coronary Care Unit at the University Hospital of South Manchester for providing other ECGs.

Appendix B, 'Ethical and legal considerations in resuscitation' by Dr Patrick Dando, was first published as 'Medico-legal problems associated with resuscitation' in the *Journal of the Medical Defence Union*, Volume 8, Numbers 1 and 2, 1992. It is reproduced here with kind permission of the Medical Defence Union and Dr Patrick Dando. All rights reserved.

The authors wish to acknowledge Karen Gwinnutt and Susan Wieteska for their assistance with preparing the text for publication.

Finally, we would like to thank the following authors who contributed to the first edition: Peter Barnes FRCP, Olive Goodall SRN, Sarah Graham MRCP, Mark James DA FRCS, Elizabeth Molyneux FRCP, Peter Nightingale MRCP FRCA, Peter Oakley MA FRCA, Richard Old, Barbara Phillips FRCP, Brian Reilly, John Shaffer MRCP, Andrew Swain PhD FRCS and David Yates MA MD MCh FRCS.

SECTION ONE
Introduction

1
Introduction

Objectives

After reading this chapter you should be able to:

- Give an overview of:

  The epidemiology and aetiology of heart disease

  The pathophysiology of heart disease

  The activities required in managing a cardiac arrest
- Understand the history of advanced cardiac life support
- Understand the aims of the book

AN OVERVIEW OF THE EPIDEMIOLOGY AND AETIOLOGY OF HEART DISEASE

The sudden cardiac event, known as a cardiac arrest, is usually the end stage of a long pathological process. In 80% of cases the patient is known to have heart disease, but in the remaining 20% of cases a cardiac arrest is the first clinical presentation.

There are many factors which contribute towards a cardiac arrest, but ischaemic heart disease is by far the most common. In the UK it is the leading cause of death in both sexes, giving rise to 82 000 male and 68 500 female deaths in 1991. These are among the highest in the world and currently cost approximately £500 million annually in treatment and £1800 million in lost production.

The American experience indicates that preventive measures can reduce the incidence of death due to cardiovascular disease. This has been taken up by the UK government, who has recently introduced a policy to try to reduce the incidence of this disease by 40% by the year 2000. Consequently, the development of advanced life support techniques should not be viewed as an excuse to continue unhealthy diets and life styles. Prevention is more effective, and much cheaper, than the present-day cure.

In contrast, in children, cardiac arrests are usually the end result of prolonged hypoxia from respiratory or circulatory failure. By the time the heart stops, other organs which are susceptible to hypoxia, such as the brain and kidneys, will also have been severely damaged. This increases the chances of the child dying from multiple organ failure should he or she survive the initial cardiac arrest. Consequently the aim in managing these patients is to recognize and treat the ill child before a cardiac arrest occurs.

AN OVERVIEW OF THE PATHOPHYSIOLOGY OF HEART DISEASE

Many factors can act alone or in combination on the myocardium to produce abnormal cardiac function (Figure 1.1), which may or may not result in the death of the muscle. In some cases effects will also be seen at other sites in the body.

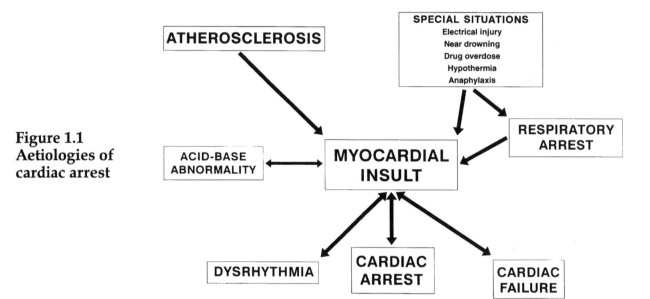

Figure 1.1 Aetiologies of cardiac arrest

The resuscitation team has to be aware of these causative factors and each of their potential end results so that the correct treatment can be provided.

THE ACTIVITIES REQUIRED IN MANAGING A CARDIAC ARREST

Most cardiac arrests occur outside hospital. Therefore, in order for the patient to survive, a whole series of activities must be carried out quickly, effectively and in the correct order.

1. Recognition
2. Commencement of basic life support techniques
3. Connecting the patient to an ECG monitor
4. Diagnosing the type of cardiac arrest rhythm

5. Rapid and early defibrillation (when appropriate)
6. Advanced life support techniques
7. Post-resuscitation care
8. Rehabilitation

This list can be depicted as the 'chain of survival' (see Figure 1.2).

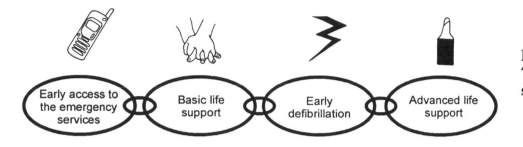

Early access to the emergency services — Basic life support — Early defibrillation — Advanced life support

Figure 1.2 The 'chain of survival'

Many studies have shown that the patient's eventual outcome is very dependent on the speed of onset and efficiency of the basic and advanced life support techniques. This was admirably demonstrated by Eisenburg's work from Seattle, which was published in the *Journal of the American Medical Association* in 1979 (Table 1.1).

Table 1.1 Incidence of survival following basic and advanced CPR

Time to CPR (min)	Time to ACLS (min)		
	<8	8–16	>16
0–4	43%	19%	10%
4–8	26%	19%	5%
8–12	–	6%	0%

It follows that ACLS is going to be of use only if effective community cardiopulmonary resuscitation (CPR) can be carried out quickly, and the patient can be defibrillated rapidly. The authors hope that the readers of this book will become involved in teaching and organising their own community CPR programmes. In that way the skills discussed can be used to greater effect.

THE HISTORY OF ADVANCED CARDIAC LIFE SUPPORT

In 1973 an advanced cardiac life support (ACLS) package was produced by the American Heart Association. Since 1980 this has been updated approximately every 5 years so that new information and changes in practice can be incorporated. Twenty three years on, tens of thousands of healthcare providers have successfully completed the ACLS course.

In 1987 the Royal College of Physicians published a report advocating the need for both basic and advanced life support training in healthcare providers. In the same year, David Skinner set up the UK's first American-style ACLS course at St Bartholomew's Hospital, London. Subsequently several centres began to run courses but the standards being taught varied. Over the following years, representatives from the various course centres were able to develop a unified course for the whole of the UK. Under the control of the Resuscitation Council (UK), the first unified course was run in January 1995.

THE AIMS OF THE BOOK

There are many ways of managing a cardiac emergency. This book aims to teach a system which is known to be both safe and effective. It will **not** train readers to be cardiologists or anaesthetists, but it **will** enable them to deal with a cardiac emergency in a logical and systematic way. In so doing it will facilitate the later management by other medical specialists.

In 1990 a group of clinicians from five acute specialties and an educationalist wrote the first edition of this book. It was based on the US Advanced Cardiac Life Support (ACLS) course manual but was modified to account for European clinicians and their way of practice. In particular, the guidelines from the European Resuscitation Council were incorporated.

Over the following 5 years more than 2000 doctors, nurses and paramedics used this book for either personnel tuition or as an ACLS course manual. Using their feedback, the authors have developed the book further so that it represents a tried and tested educational package relevant for all healthcare personnel working in the acute sector. It is important to realize, however, that the knowledge gained is aimed at enhancing, not replacing, the in-house training that personnel already receive in their own hospitals or institutions.

The material is presented in a didactic fashion. Some of the latest therapeutic programmes and concepts have not been included, either because they are not universally available or because they are not generally accepted.

2

The natural history of myocardial infarction

Objectives

After reading this chapter you should be able to:

- Understand the epidemiology and pathophysiology of myocardial infarction

- Understand how to diagnose myocardial infarction

- Understand the principles of the immediate management of myocardial infarction

---

INTRODUCTION

Myocardial infarction (MI) is one manifestation of a spectrum of conditions referred to as ischaemic heart disease. This also includes silent myocardial ischaemia, stable and unstable angina pectoris and sudden cardiac death. All, however, have a common under-lying pathology – coronary artery atheroma.

Acute myocardial infarction is defined as myocardial necrosis due to cessation of, or interference with, the blood supply. Macroscopic evidence of myocardial infarction may be either regional, when related to thrombosis in the supplying artery, or global, secondary to an overall reduction in myocardial perfusion, e.g. extensive atheromatous disease and cardiogenic shock.

EPIDEMIOLOGY OF MYOCARDIAL INFARCTION

Current mortality rates following myocardial infarction vary both between countries and within each country. Unfortunately, the mortality rates in the UK are amongst the highest in the world, at approximately 250 per 100 000 for men and women aged 30–69 years. Furthermore there is close correlation between the relative mortality rates of men and women; however, the incidence in males is greater than females by approximately a ratio of 3:1. There is a decline in chronic mortality in western countries. These changes are most evident in the younger age groups, with an approximate 50% reduction since 1969 in both males and females aged 35–49 years. Unfortunately mortality in Eastern Europe is increasing.

Risk factors for ischaemic heart disease include increased age, male sex, cigarette smoking, family history of ischaemic heart disease, hypertension, hyperlipidaemia (in particular hypercholesterol-aemia), diabetes, and obesity. A recent health survey of England showed the following disappointing facts:

- Approximately one-third of the population continue to smoke.
- Almost one in five adults are hypertensive.
- 70% have cholesterol levels above the desirable values.
- More than half are overweight or obese.

Hence, there is still considerable scope for primary and secondary prevention of ischaemic heart disease.

PATHOPHYSIOLOGY

Atherosclerosis is a disease of large- and medium-sized blood vessels. Crucial changes take place in the lining of the artery (the intima) through which lipids (cholesterol in particular) penetrate the endothelium. Subsequently collagen and calcium are laid down in the blood vessel wall, changing its integrity and elasticity, the overall effect being to produce luminal narrowing and as a consequence a reduction in blood supply (Figure 2.1).

A trigger to the formation of atherosclerosis is believed to be injury to the vascular endothelium. Hyperlipidaemia, cigarette smoking and systemic hypertension may be implicated in producing endothelial damage or dysfunction. The consequent increase in permeability will facilitate adhesion of platelets and monocytes to exposed subendothelial cells. As a part of this interaction a variety of potent pro-inflammatory compounds are released which will stimulate the development of smooth muscle cells and a lipid collagen matrix.

Early changes like these may be seen even in infants and teenagers. They are often referred to as 'fatty streaks'. In contrast, the atherosclerotic lesions in adults occur as plaques surrounded by a fibrous tissue. These plaques can cause concentric or eccentric narrowing of the blood vessel lumen. Concentric plaques in particular often reflect extensive involvement of the underlying media (Figure 2.1).

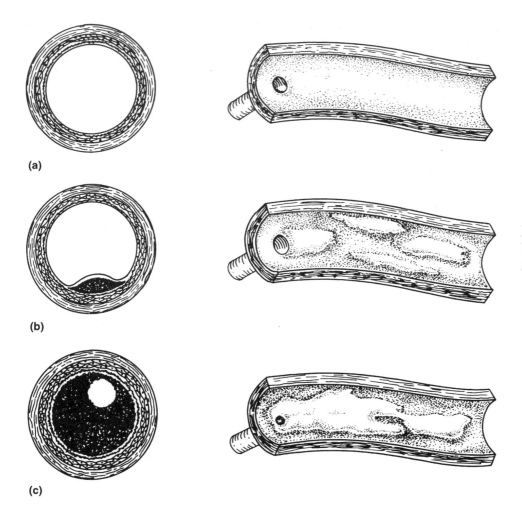

**Figure 2.1
Development of
atheroma**

Plaques are fundamental to the development of angina, acute MI and sudden ischaemic death. In all three instances a thrombus can be found within the coronary artery. Two mechanisms are responsible for producing thrombus in the coronary arteries and both involve injury to the intima (Figure 2.2). The first mechanism, superficial intimal injury, causes denudation of the endothelium, but the atheromatous plaque remains intact. The second mechanism, deep intimal injury, is common and a tear or fissure occurs within the plaque. Irrespective of the mechanism intimal injury occurs, resulting in exposure of subendothelial collagen. Platelets adhere to it, leading to the production of thrombin and fibrin with subsequent formation of a fibrin mesh. This mesh stabilizes the platelet thrombus, which is firmly fixed to the wall.

The formation of thrombus in this fashion is the first step in the process of thrombosis. As it grows or propagates it may protrude into and finally occlude the arterial lumen. It is important to realize, however, that the thrombus can also be reabsorbed or recanalized.

Figure 2.2 Thrombus formation

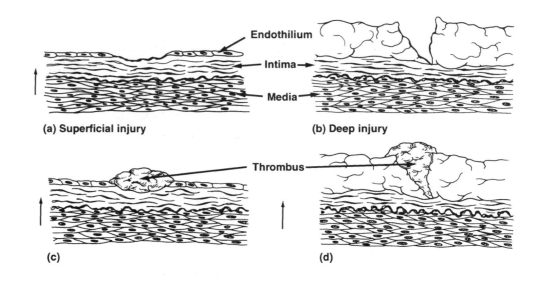

(a) Superficial injury   (b) Deep injury

(c)   (d)

Endothilium
Intima
Media
Thrombus

CLINICAL RECOGNITION OF MYOCARDIAL INFARCTION

Most patients suffering an MI will experience severe chest pain, the characteristics of which are well known. However, it is worth emphasizing that pain can occur at remote sites, e.g. epigastric pain may indicate an inferior myocardial infarction, whereas shoulder or even wrist pain may indicate acute coronary ischaemia. Such symptoms, if lasting more than 30 min, should alert the physician to a possible underlying myocardial infarct.

Often there are no abnormal physical findings. However, the clinical picture may be dominated by autonomic activity, in particular sweating, peripheral vasoconstriction, tachycardia and pallor. Vomiting may be a reflection of extreme pain or vagal activity.

Early diagnosis of myocardial infarction

The electrocardiogram (ECG)

A 12-lead electrocardiogram (ECG) is invaluable in the diagnosis of MI. However, it is important to realize that the classical ECG changes of ST elevation, T wave inversion and Q wave formation may not be evident when the patient first presents. Thus a patient who is suspected of having either unstable angina or MI should have repeated electrocardiograms every 15–30 min because diagnostic changes may suddenly occur. A normal ECG does not exclude the diagnosis of MI. The ECG is also of benefit in that it will delineate the site of infarction and provide information underlying associated dysrhythmias (Figure 2.3).

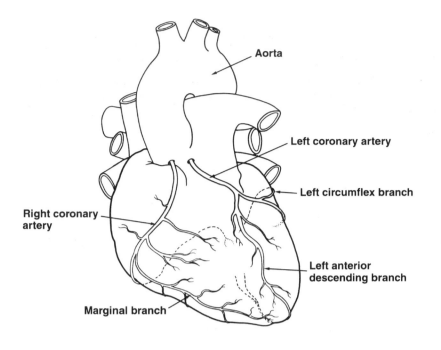

Figure 2.3   The coronary arteries

Cardiac enzymes

Measurement of two cardiac enzymes, creatine kinase and hydroxy-butyrate dehydrogenase, are used to confirm the diagnosis of MI. Unfortunately, even a rapid rise of creatine kinase (CK) or its more cardiospecific isoenzyme (CKMB) within 4–8 h is not early enough to allow intervention to be deferred until cardiac enzyme results are available. Serum aspartate transaminase (AST) has a similar release profile to CK but unfortunately is not as specific as it is released from many other tissues.

Hydroxybutyrate dehydrogenase (HBD) is used as an indicator of lactate dehydrogenase 1 (LDH_1) activity, and is more cardiospecific than AST. Unfortunately, it may take 12–24 h before it is detectable and, more importantly, it may be released from the lung in heart failure. However, HBD is useful in confirming MI in patients who present some days after their chest pain as it remains elevated for 7–12 days after infarct.

Other markers of myocardial damage include myoglobin, which is released within 60–90 min, but unfortunately it may also be released from skeletal muscle and a single sample, if negative, does not indicate that an MI has not occurred.

More sensitive and specific markers of myocardial necrosis are being developed – such as troponin T (a subunit of muscle binding protein). This rises slightly later than myoglobin and is virtually 100% specific.

To diagnose MI, two criteria from the following list are required:

1. A history of chest pain of greater than 30 min duration.
2. Evidence of ST elevation greater than 1 mm in two adjacent leads, the presence of new Q waves or persistent ST depression in V1–V3 with tall r waves (suggestive of an acute posterior infarction).
3. Cardiac enzyme levels (CKMB, HBD) greater than twice the upper limit.

MANAGEMENT

Initial management

Oxygen should be administered in all cases and adequate analgesia is mandatory. The latter will have the direct effect of reducing chest pain and anxiety as well as an indirect beneficial effect on catecholamine secretion. Enhanced catecholamine secretion may increase the risk of a rhythm disturbance and the size of the MI. Most patients will require intravenous opiates, usually diamorphine, which should always be accompanied by an anti-emetic. Occasionally, however, buccal or sublingual nitrates are sufficient. The administration of analgesia should be governed by the frequency and severity of pain.

Oral aspirin should be given immediately to all patients with a suspected diagnosis of MI, especially as there is little associated risk in the event of a misdiagnosis. Do not forget that aspirin has a beneficial effect on outcome following MI. Furthermore, this effect is additive to that of thrombolysis.

At the onset of symptoms the patient is at high risk, in pain and usually not at the hospital. Resuscitation facilities will be available only when paramedical staff arrive and the patient should be transferred quickly to the hospital. Unless the patient is seen by a general practitioner many of the above drugs are not available out of hospital. A useful substitute is Entonox (a 50:50 mixture of oxygen and nitrous oxide) which can be administered via a patient controlled device.

Once the patient has reached hospital specific treatment can be given to optimize outcome. Some authorities, however, would favour administration of thrombolytics before the patient reaches hospital.

Thrombolysis

Thrombolytics limit the damage associated with MI and have had a substantial effect in reducing mortality. Early administration is mandatory as ischaemic death is a rapid process. The choice of thrombolytic is less important than ensuring rapid administration. If given within 2 h of coronary occlusion mortality is considerably reduced. There is still a beneficial effect for up to 24 h after infarction, although this is less marked.

There are currently three main thrombolytic agents – streptokinase, recombinant tissue plasminogen activator (rTPA; Alteplase) and anisoylated plasminogen activator complex (Apsac; anistreplase). The details of these three agents are considered in Chapter 3.

Many studies (e.g. ISIS 3, GISSI 2) have shown that there is little difference in benefit between these thrombolytic agents. More recently, an accelerated TPA regimen has been shown to have a more favourable outcome than streptokinase (GUSTO trial). This, however, must be viewed in the light of greater costs, a high incidence of haemorrhagic strokes, especially in those over 75 years, and a skewed population with regard to the treatment time for thrombolysis. It is important to realize that MI is more common in the elderly and is associated with a higher mortality. Nevertheless, increasing age is **not** a contraindication for thrombolysis despite the increased risk of bleeding.

Although there is little to choose between thrombolytic agents, it would appear that most patients still receive streptokinase. Tissue plasminogen activator is given to patients who have had recurrent infarction or who have been given streptokinase between 5 days and 12 months previously. The accelerated TPA regimen is reserved, by most people, for patients who have a low risk of stroke (usually under 55 years of age and systolic blood pressure of less than 140 mmHg), and who present within 3 h of the onset of their symptoms. Intravenous heparin is usually co-administered with TPA.

Thrombolytic therapy should be administered only when there are diagnostic ECG changes, i.e. at least 2 mm of ST segment elevation in two consecutive anterior precordial leads or 1 mm of ST elevation in two standard limb leads.

Beta-blockers

The benefit of beta blockade following myocardial infarction was proven in the ISIS-1 trial before the thrombolytic era, but unfortunately these agents appear to be rarely used. Beta blockade has been shown to prevent one cardiac arrest, one reinfarction and one death in approximately every 200 patients. The improved survival is achieved by preventing death from cardiac rupture within the first 24 h. Atenolol or metoprolol should be given intravenously initially, followed by an oral maintenance dose. Metoprolol has the advantage of having a short half-life. All patients without contraindication (see Chapter 3) should be treated with intravenous beta-blockade within the first 24 h and maintained on oral therapy for at least one year.

Other drugs

Nitrates

Unfortunately, although several studies have suggested some benefit, no single study has actually demonstrated this.

Angiotensin-converting enzyme (ACE) inhibitors

Following MI, ventricular remodelling occurs as a result of structural changes in the composition and thickness of the ventricular wall and the chamber size. These can affect left ventricular function which is a major determinant of outcome following MI. ACE inhibitors have a beneficial effect on remodelling by limiting infarct expansion and preventing ventricular dilatation.

There are still many unanswered questions regarding ACE inhibitors in this context, in particular how soon after infarction the inhibitors should be started. Overall these drugs reduce mortality, and the patients who benefit are those who have had a recent myocardial infarction that is large and has resulted in left ventricular dysfunction, heart failure, chronic left ventricular dysfunction or chronic heart failure.

Calcium antagonists

The role of calcium channel antagonists following MI is still open to debate. Oral nifedipine has failed to produce any benefit and an adverse trend in mortality has been noted. In contrast, diltiazem has been shown to reduce mortality but only in patients with non-'Q' wave infarction. Furthermore, it has been shown to reduce mortality in patients without heart failure, but to increase mortality in those with heart failure.

Magnesium

This has proven to be beneficial in the treatment of certain ventricular arrhythmias. Magnesium also induces vasodilatation but its use in limiting infarct size is questionable. Although the ISIS 4 trial did not show any benefit with magnesium, local policies may vary regarding its use.

POST-INFARCT COMPLICATIONS

A variety of complications are seen in patients following myocardial infarction:

- Left ventricular/biventricular failure
- Dysrhythmias
- Mitral valve dysfunction
- Mural thrombus
- Septal rupture
- Pericardial tamponade
- Systemic/pulmonary emboli

These can result in a range of complications, from death to severe disability, secondary to decreased cardiac function.

PSYCHOLOGICAL ASPECTS OF MYOCARDIAL INFARCTION

The psychological impact of MI upon the patient and the relatives is high. Anxiety and chest pain increase both catecholamine levels and the risk of rhythm disturbance. Reassurance and analgesia are therefore important. It is also important to remember that on admission the patient has usually already survived the greatest period of risk.

Under ideal circumstances all patients with suspected MI should be admitted to a coronary care unit. This, however, is unlikely, and important aspects of initial management are likely to occur out in the pre-hospital environment, in the emergency department and intensive care unit. Lack of communication is often a problem and seriously undermines the patient's and relatives' confidence. Close liaison between all people involved in the patient's management is essential. The initial management should be seen as the first step in the process of rehabilitation.

SUMMARY

MI is a common condition. Although the incidence in the Western world is falling, advice on prevention is often unheeded. The diagnosis of MI is based on the patient's history, changes on the ECG and cardiac enzyme release. Although the management of such patients may vary all should receive oxygen, aspirin, analgesic and thrombolysis.

REFERENCES

ISIS-1: Randomised trial of intravenous atenolol among 16,027 cases of suspected acute myocardial infarction: ISIS-1. First International Study of Infarct Survival Collaborative Group. *Lancet.* Jul 12 1986; **2**:(8498) 57–66.

ISIS-3: A randomised comparison of streptokinase vs tissue plasminogen activator vs anistreplase and of aspirin plus heparin vs aspirin alone among 41,299 cases of suspected acute myocardial infarction. ISIS-3 (Third International Study of Infarct Survival) Collaborative Group. *Lancet.* 1992; **339**: 753–770.

ISIS-4: A randomised factorial trial assessing early oral captopril, oral mononitrate, and intravenous magnesium sulphate in 58,050 patients with suspected acute myocardial infarction. ISIS-4 (Fourth International Study of Infarct Survival) Collaborative Group. *Lancet.* 1995; **345**: 669–685.

GUSTO: An international trial comparing four thrombolytic strategies for acute myocardial infarction. The GUSTO investigators. *N. Engl. J. Med.* 1993; **329**: 673–682.

GISSI-2: A factorial randomised trial of alteplase versus streptokinase and heparin versus no heparin among 12,490 patients with acute myocardial infarction. Gruppo Italiano per lo Studio della Sopravvivenza nell'Infarcto Miocardico. *Lancet.* 1990; **336**: 65–71.

——— 3 ———
Pharmacology

Objectives

After reading this chapter you should be able to:

- Understand the actions, indications and dosages of drugs used in cardiac resuscitation
- Understand the special precautions and contraindications for drugs used in cardiac resuscitation

INTRODUCTION

This chapter describes drugs used in the management of myocardial infarction, cardiac arrests and arrhythmias. However, many of the drugs are used in more than one of these situations. The list below is only an arbitrary classification of the drugs considered in this chapter.

Drugs used for myocardial infarction

Aspirin
Inotropic agents
Naloxone
Nitrates
Opioids
Thrombolytics

Drugs for cardiac arrest

Adrenaline
Atropine
Bretylium
Calcium
Lignocaine
Sodium bicarbonate

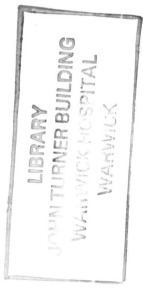

Drugs for arrhythmias

Adenosine
Amiodarone
Atenolol (see beta-blockers)
Beta-blockers
Digoxin
Esmolol (see beta-blockers)
Isoprenaline
Magnesium
Verapamil

Some of the terms used in this chapter are not comprehensively explained. However, their meanings will become clear as you continue to read this book.

Rather than try to read this chapter from start to finish, you may find it of more educational benefit (and easier to learn) if it is used for reference – when a drug is mentioned in the book refer to this chapter for comprehensive details. To ensure ease of reference the drugs have been considered in alphabetical order. Many of the anti-arrhythmic drugs are classified according to their mechanism of action. One such classification is shown in Table 3.1.

Table 3.1 The Vaughan-Williams Singh classification of anti-arrhythmic drugs

Class	Action
I	Local anaesthetic drugs which diminish membrane responsiveness and conductivity by reducing sodium ion flux into the cells
IA	Usually prolong repolarization
IB	Usually shorten repolarization
IC	Little effect on repolarization
II	Antagonize the effects of catecholamines without direct effects on cardiac tissue. Beta-adrenergic blockade
III	Prolong the action potential without affecting membrane responsiveness
IV	Calcium-channel blockade

It is important to remember that:

Drugs that can treat arrhythmias can cause arrhythmias.

INDIVIDUAL DRUGS

Adenosine

Indications:

Paroxysmal supraventricular tachycardia (PSVT)

Undiagnosed wide complex tachycardia

The initial dose is 3 mg, given rapidly by injection into a large vein, followed by a saline flush. Repeated doses, after 1–2 min, of 6 mg, 12 mg and 18 mg may be given. The injection must be fast to achieve adequate and effective blood levels as the half-life of adenosine is only 10–15 s.

Adenosine should be used only in a monitored environment, e.g. in the coronary care unit (CCU), intensive care unit (ICU) or the emergency department.

Adenosine is a naturally occurring purine nucleotide. It is a class IV anti-arrhythmic agent that slows conduction across the atrioventricular node (A-V node) but has little effect on other myocardial cells. This action makes it highly effective for terminating PSVT with re-entrant circuits that include the A-V node (see Chapter 8). This effect, however, may be temporary because of the drug's short duration of action. Adenosine-induced A-V nodal block may, in patients with a narrow complex tachycardia, reveal the underlying atrial tachycardia by slowing the ventricular response.

The major advantage of adenosine is that, unlike verapamil, it can be given to a patient with a broad complex tachycardia of uncertain aetiology. The ventricular response in a supraventricular tachycardia (SVT) will be slowed, junctional tachycardias will be terminated, but a ventricular tachycardia (VT) will continue unchanged. Another advantage is that adenosine does not cause significant negative inotropic effects, i.e. decrease in ventricular contractility resulting in reduced cardiac output and low blood pressure. Adenosine can also be given safely to a patient who is on beta-blockers.

Administration of adenosine is associated with a wide variety of 'strange feelings' which may include severe chest pain. Patients should be warned to expect these and be reassured that they will settle very quickly without further treatment. This drug may also induce or worsen bronchospasm in patients who have asthma.

The effects of adenosine are enhanced by dipyridamole and antagonized by theophylline.

Adrenaline (epinephrine)

Indications:

Promote cerebral and coronary blood flow. (First drug in each of the cardiac arrest protocols.)

In cardiac arrest the intravenous dose is 1 mg initially or 2–3 mg via the endotracheal tube (where appropriate, and where venous access is delayed or cannot be achieved). The 1 mg dose is repeated every 3 min until resuscitation is either successful or abandoned.

Adrenaline is available in two dilutions, 1 in 1000 (1 g in 1000 ml) and 1 in 10 000 (1 g in 10 000 ml). Thus 1 mg is contained in 1 ml of 1:1000 or 10 ml of 10 000. The 1 in 10 000 dilution is commonly used in cardiac resuscitation.

Adrenaline, a naturally occurring catecholamine, acts as a neurotransmitter in the sympathetic nervous system possessing both α- and β-adrenergic effects. The α effects result in arteriolar vasoconstriction and an increase in peripheral vascular resistance. The overall effect of this in cardiac arrest is to 'divert' blood flow to the brain and heart. The β effects are mediated by β_1 and β_2 receptors. Stimulation of β_1 receptors increases heart rate (a chronotropic effect) and contraction force (an inotropic effect). Stimulation of β_2 receptors produces bronchodilation. The β_1-mediated effects are potentially harmful as they increase the oxygen requirement of the myocardium, which can either induce or increase ischaemia.

Adrenaline increases myocardial excitability and is therefore arrhythmogenic, especially when the myocardium is ischaemic and/or hypoxic. These effects, however, are not relevant to either the cardiac arrest situation or immediate post-resuscitation care.

Amiodarone

Indications:

All resistant arrhythmias

Wolff–Parkinson–White syndrome

A loading dose of 300 mg in 100 ml 5% dextrose (not saline) is given over 15 min followed by a further 300 mg over 1 h. The maximum dose is 1.2 g in 24 h. It can then be given orally for 5–10 days, e.g. 200 mg daily.

Amiodarone is a class III anti-arrhythmic agent because it increases the duration of the action potential in atrial and ventricular myocardium. Thus, it prolongs the PR and QT intervals. It also has some class I activity, inhibiting fast sodium channels. In addition, amiodarone may exhibit non-competitive α-blocking effects and mild negative inotropic effects when given intravenously and coronary artery vasodilatation when given orally. If given concurrently with other drugs which act to prolong the QT interval (e.g. local anaesthetic agents) amiodarone may 'paradoxically' become pro-arrhythmogenic.

The effects of warfarin and digoxin are potentiated by amiodarone, therefore their doses should be reduced by approximately half. Amiodarone also has an additive effect with beta-blockers and calcium channel blockers, resulting in an increased degree of nodal block.

Most of the side effects of amiodarone are not relevant to emergency treatment, although nausea is common, even at low doses. Other side effects occur after prolonged administration, e.g. photosensitivity, 'blue-grey' skin discoloration, abnormalities of thyroid function, corneal microdeposits, peripheral neuropathy and pulmonary infiltrates.

Aspirin

Indications:

Unstable angina to prevent infarction

Anti-thrombotic effect in myocardial infarction

Secondary prophylaxis post myocardial infarction

The actions of aspirin depend on the dose given. This varies between 75 mg and >3 g/day. Lower doses can be tried for people who are normally intolerant of aspirin.

1. Anti-thrombotic effects are achieved by low-dose treatment, i.e. 75–325 mg/day, which interferes with platelet thromboxane A synthesis and reduces 'stickiness'.
2. Analgesic effects are achieved by moderate doses, 1–3 g/day.
3. Non-steroidal anti-inflammatory effects are achieved at high doses (3 g/day or more). However, aspirin becomes prothrombotic at these levels (by diminishing prostacyclin formation).

Aspirin reduces mortality following myocardial infarction. When combined with streptokinase a greater reduction in mortality occurs – as clearly demonstrated in the ISIS 2 trial.

The adverse effects associated with aspirin, i.e. gastrointestinal bleeding and possible exacerbation of peptic ulcers, are rare and insignificant at low, anti-thrombotic, doses. However, in susceptible individuals, low-dose aspirin can precipitate an acute attack of gout!

Atropine

Indications:

Asystole

Bradycardia with risk of asystole, or adverse signs

The recommended adult dose for asystole is 3 mg IV. Although 6 mg may be given by the endotracheal route this is not advocated because of the large volume of fluid that is administered. For the treatment of symptomatic bradycardia, an initial dose of 0.5–1 mg IV is required. Repeated doses may be necessary for or during pacemaker insertion.

Atropine competes with the parasympathetic neurotransmitter acetylcholine at muscarinic receptors. Hence its cardiac effects are mediated by vagal inhibition at the level of the sino-atrial node (SAN) and A-V node. This increases heart rate and (rate-related) cardiac output. The blood pressure may also rise as a secondary phenomenon.

Parasympathetic nervous stimulation by the vagus nerve can result in a bradycardia, which may respond to atropine. Unfortunately there is no conclusive evidence, only anecdotal reports, that atropine is beneficial in asystole. In view of the poor prognosis from this condition atropine may be useful and, possibly more importantly, is unlikely to be harmful.

Side effects of atropine become more prominent as the dose increases but they are not relevant to the cardiac arrest situation. Note that dilated pupils in a post-arrest patient should not be attributed solely to the use of atropine. Following IV administration, anticholinergic side effects may occur – in particular, blurred vision, dry mouth, urinary retention and acute confusional states.

Beta-blockers

Indications:

Unstable angina

Second-line treatment for supraventricular tachycardia (SVT) when no adverse signs

The beneficial effects of beta-blockers after myocardial infarction, especially in the treatment of tachycardia with persistent hypertension and/or ventricular arrhythmias, was clearly shown in the ISIS 1 trial (see Chapter 2).

There are numerous types of beta-blocking drugs with different dosages and proportions of β_1 to β_2 antagonist activity.

Non-selective beta-blockers

These agents, e.g. propranolol, non-selectively block β_1 and β_2 receptors to reduce heart rate by a combination of circulating catecholamine antagonism and reduction of A-V node conduction. The dose for treatment of an SVT is 1 mg IV, repeated once if necessary. They have a negative inotropic effect, i.e. they reduce cardiac contractility. Antagonism of bronchiolar β_2 receptors may lead to significant bronchospasm in susceptible individuals. The half-life of propranolol is 4 h.

Esmolol is an alternative drug which has a very short half life (8 min) and is therefore ideal for the treatment of an SVT. Initial IV dose is 500 μg/kg given over 1 min followed by an infusion of 50 μg/kg per min.

Second-generation agents

These are relatively cardioselective, i.e. block β_1 receptors almost exclusively, although this benefit is lost at high doses. An example is atenolol and the usual oral dose is 50–100 mg/day.

Third-generation agents

These agents, e.g. Celiprolol, are relatively cardioselective. They also have some vasodilatory properties mediated through partial agonist activity on β_2 receptors in arterial vessel walls.

It is important to realize that the use of any beta-blocker may precipitate left ventricular failure in patients with an already failing ventricle, hypotension, or heart block. Profound bradycardia may develop and may be difficult to treat. The risk of heart block or asystole is increased if IV verapamil is co-administered, especially if the beta-blocker was also given intravenously. For similar reasons, the combination of beta-blockers and class I anti-arrhythmic agents should be avoided. Thus, care is required in the treatment of SVT to avoid converting a non-life-threatening condition into a life-threatening condition by injudicious polypharmacy.

Bretylium tosylate

Indications:

Refractory ventricular tachycardia (VT)

Ventricular fibrillation (VF)

Bretylium is administered intravenously. The initial dose is 5 mg/kg and may be increased to 10 mg/kg for refractory ventricular arrhythmias. If successful this should be followed by an infusion of 1–2 mg/kg per h. The maximum daily dose should not exceed 30 mg/kg.

The anti-arrhythmic actions of Bretylium are poorly understood. It is currently described as a class III anti-arrhythmic agent acting mainly on Purkinje fibres and less on ventricular muscle. It is taken up by terminal sympathetic neurons and initially causes the release of stored noradrenaline which in turn may transiently cause a deterioration in the rhythm and hypotension. Bretylium is stored in the nerve terminals and because it prevents further neurotransmitter release it is said to cause a 'chemical sympathectomy'. The half-life is 13–15 h.

It is likely that the antiarrhythmic properties of Bretylium are unrelated to this adrenergic effect. However, Bretylium does increase the threshold for ventricular fibrillation.

Bretylium may take up to 30 min to achieve its effect and so use of this drug in a cardiac arrest commits the resuscitation team to continuing basic life support for at least 30 min after administration.

The major troublesome side effects are nausea and hypotension and the latter may necessitate plasma volume expansion. Bretylium should not be given by the intra-osseous route.

Calcium

Indications:

Electromechanical dissociation (after adrenaline) caused by:

  severe hyperkalaemia
  severe hypocalcaemia
  overdose of Ca^{2+} channel blockers

The initial dose of 10 ml of 10% calcium chloride (13.6 mmol Ca^{2+}) or gluconate is recommended (calcium chloride solutions contain approximately twice the concentration of calcium when compared with calcium gluconate solutions).

Calcium assists in muscle contraction. *In vitro*, calcium will not only restart an arrested heart preparation but will also cause marked cerebral and coronary artery vasospasm. Similarly, *in vivo* high plasma concentrations of calcium may have detrimental effects on the ischaemic myocardium and cerebral function – in particular after a cardiac arrest. Thus calcium is given only during cardiac resuscitation when a specific indication is present or strongly suspected.

Calcium chloride should not be given immediately before or after sodium bicarbonate without first flushing the line. This prevents precipitation within the IV line or the cannula.

Digoxin toxicity is aggravated by a high serum calcium.

Digoxin

Indications:

Atrial fibrillation with fast ventricular response

Left ventricular failure

Rapid digitalization can be achieved by either IV administration or a combination of IV and oral loading doses. A dose of 0.5 mg digoxin in 50 ml 5% dextrose is given IV over 1 h followed by 0.25 mg orally once or twice until 0.75 mg or 1.0 mg has been given in 24 h. If the patient is small, old or frail, a lower loading dose must be used. Oral maintenance doses usually lie between 0.0625 mg and 0.5 mg per day.

Digoxin is a cardiac glycoside which slows the ventricular rate by increasing vagal tone, decreasing sympathetic drive and increasing the refractory period in the A-V node. It also enhances myocardial contractility and decreases conduction velocity in the Purkinje fibres. The half-life is 36 h.

Side effects increase in severity as the serum levels rise. They include nausea, diarrhoea, anorexia, confusion and dizziness. A wide variety of arrhythmias may also develop, ranging from atrial tachycardia with varying degrees of block to ventricular extrasystoles and bigemini. Digoxin toxicity can be confirmed by direct measurement of blood levels. Toxicity is increased by hypokalaemia, hypomagnesaemia, hypoxia, hypercalcaemia, renal failure or hypothyroidism.

See Chapter 13 for the treatment of digoxin toxicity.

Frusemide

Indications:

Left ventricular failure (LVF)

Congestive cardiac failure

The adult dose required varies from 20 mg to 120 mg IV.

Frusemide is a diuretic which acts on the ascending limb of the loop of Henle in the kidney to produce a diuresis within 10–20 min of an intravenous injection. It is more powerful than thiazide diuretics and can produce a response even when the glomerular filtration rate is low. Another important action is venodilatation with a consequent reduction in myocardial preload. This precedes the diuretic action and explains why a patient with acute pulmonary oedema secondary to LVF feels less breathless even before the diuresis has occurred.

As long as hypotension and/or hypovolaemia have been excluded, anuria is not a contraindication to the use of frusemide. Hypokalaemia may develop during treatment and may precipitate arrhythmias, especially when used either early after MI or when the patient has been digitalized. Therefore careful attention must be given to IV or oral potassium replacement (noting that an adult requires 40–80 mmol potassium per day) or co-prescription of a potassium-sparing diuretic.

Inotropic agents

Rational use of inotropic agents requires the use of invasive monitoring since their actions may be unpredictable. They should be administered via a catheter in a central vein.

Dopamine

Indications:

Hypotension not due to hypovolaemia

To promote a diuresis

The usual starting dose is 2 μg/kg/min (via an infusion pump) and increased as necessary to achieve the desired effect. Invasive monitoring is advocated.

Dopamine is the precursor of the naturally occurring catecholamines adrenaline and noradrenaline. It has a positive inotropic effect that is mediated by dopamine (D_1 and D_2 receptors), as well as α_1, α_2 and β_1 receptors of the sympathetic nervous system. The effects of dopamine are dose dependent.

At low infusion rates (1–2 μg/kg/min) renal vasodilatation occurs (via D_1 receptors) resulting in increased glomerular filtration rate and sodium excretion. Intermediate infusion rates (2–10 μg/kg/min) increase cardiac output, systolic blood pressure and renal responses – mediated via β_1 receptors. At the highest infusion rates (>10 μg/kg/min) α_1 and α_2 receptors are stimulated. Ventricular filling pressures and the peripheral resistance are increased, resulting in an increased myocardial oxygen demand, which is detrimental to the failing heart.

Dopamine has the potential to increase myocardial oxygen demand beyond the supply. Thus it may be arrhythmogenic, worsen ischaemia and may even increase the size of an infarct.

Side effects include headache, nausea and vomiting. Extravasation at the site of the IV cannula may produce tissue damage. Hypotension may result if the drug is either co-prescribed with phenytoin or abruptly withdrawn. Hypertensive crisis can occur in patients taking monoamine oxidase inhibitors.

Inotropes such as dopamine impair the utero-placental circulation, rendering the fetus hypoxic and therefore in jeopardy. Thus dopamine should be used in pregnant women **only** when the expected benefits outweigh the potential risk to the fetus.

Dobutamine

Indications:

Hypotension not due to hypovolaemia

Cardiogenic shock.

The dose starts at 2.5 μg/kg/min and is increased gradually, until the desired effect is achieved. Invasive monitoring is essential.

Dobutamine is a synthetic catecholamine with stimulating properties mediated by β_1, β_2 and α_1 receptors. Major effects of dopamine are to increase the rate and force of contraction. The resultant increase in cardiac output and hence renal blood flow results in diuresis. Its advantage over dopamine is that it tends to lower cardiac filling pressures and usually the peripheral vascular resistance. It has a similar potential for increasing myocardial oxygen demand beyond supply, increasing infarct size and inducing arrhythmias.

Isoprenaline

Indications:

Symptomatic bradycardia, unresponsive to atropine

If 2 mg isoprenaline is mixed in 500 ml 5% dextrose, a 4 μg/ml solution results. This is infused at 2–10 μg/min (i.e. 0.5–2.5 ml/min). The half-life is approximately 2 min.

Isoprenaline is a sympathomimetic amine with almost pure β_1 and β_2 agonist, and virtually no α activity. It is more chronotropic than inotropic (β_1 effects) and also reduces peripheral vascular resistance by dilating vessels in the splanchnic circulation and skeletal muscle (β_2 effects). It is used as an interim treatment only to augment the action of atropine providing haemodynamic support before transvenous cardiac pacing.

As with other inotropes isoprenaline may increase myocardial oxygen demands, infarct size and the risk of tachyarrhythmias.

Lignocaine (lidocaine)

Indications:

Haemodynamically stable ventricular tachycardia (VT)

Refractory ventricular fibrillation (VF)

An initial rapid IV dose, either 100 mg for VF or 50 mg for haemo-dynamically stable VT, given over 2 min. This may be repeated every 5 min up to 200 mg or the first dose can be followed by an infusion of 2 mg/min.

Lignocaine is classified as a 1B antiarrhythmic agent, because it inhibits the fast sodium current and shortens the duration of the action potential. It acts selectively in diseased and ischaemic tissue by interrupting and preventing re-entry circuits. As lignocaine stabilizes cell membranes it suppresses ventricular premature extrasystole, and is a good local anaesthetic.

Lignocaine is metabolized very rapidly by the liver and should be used with caution in patients with hepatic impairment. For arrhythmia management it must be given intravenously. An initial dose of 50 mg is rapidly distributed throughout the body and is effective for approximately 10 min. It must be followed by a second dose of 100 mg, and then an infusion of 2–4 mg/min. The half-life is then prolonged (2 h) unless the hepatic blood flow is reduced. However, during cardiac arrest normal clearance mechanisms do not function and high plasma concentrations may exist after a single dose. Lignocaine is less effective in the presence of hypokalaemia and hypomagnesaemia.

In general, the severity of symptoms and signs of lignocaine toxicity are dependent on the speed of infusion or rapidity of absorption rather than the plasma concentration.

At higher rates of infusion, the patient may feel dizzy, notice difficulty in speaking, numbness around the mouth or become drowsy. If blood levels rise further convulsions occur and death ensues. Even when using lignocaine as a local anaesthetic it is worth remembering that the currently accepted maximum safe dose in a healthy person is 3 mg/kg.

Magnesium sulphate

Indications:

Broad complex tachycardia, including torsades des pointes, with hypokalaemia.

The initial dose is 8 mmol (4 ml of 50%), intravenously, which may be repeated after 10–15 min.

Magnesium is an important constituent of many enzyme systems, especially those involved with energy generation in muscle. It is also essential for neurochemical transmission where it decreases acetylcholine release and reduces the sensitivity of the motor end plate. Therefore excess magnesium will depress neurological and myocardial function by acting as a physiological calcium blocker – like potassium.

Intravenous magnesium is a safe and effective treatment in broad complex tachycardias. The role of magnesium in acute myocardial infarction is still unproven. As hypokalaemic patients are often hypomagnesaemic the two are frequently administered concurrently.

Magnesium is excreted by the kidneys, but side effects associated with hypermagnesaemia are rare even in renal failure.

Naloxone

Indications:

Opioid overdose

Naloxone is a specific competitive antagonist at μ and κ opiate receptors. It will reverse all the effects of exogenous opioids, in particular cerebral and respiratory depression. The duration of action is very short and repeated injections are often required.

Adults need an initial dose of 0.8–2 mg IV. This may be repeated every 2–3 min if necessary, to a maximum of 10 mg. Alternatively, an infusion can be used, adjusting the rate to achieve the desired effect.

Side effects following naloxone administration are rare.

Nitrates

Indications:

Prophylaxis/relief of angina

Unstable angina

Acute myocardial infarction

Left ventricular failure (LVF) (acute and chronic)

The dose depends upon the nitrate used and route of administration.

There are several routes of administration for nitrates: transdermal, buccal and sublingual, oral and intravenous infusion. Nitrates delivered via the buccal and sublingual routes are useful in the acute situation as they are effective within 1–2 min. If side effects occur, they can be easily and rapidly stopped by removing the tablet. Although sublingual GTN spray (0.4 mg metered dose) used twice is very effective it has the disadvantage that the dose cannot be adjusted if the patient becomes hypotensive.

Nitrates cause vascular smooth muscle relaxation by conversion to nitric oxide (NO). This dilatation is more marked on the venous than the arterial side of the circulation, so that myocardial preload is reduced proportionately more than afterload. Nitrates also dilate the coronary arteries, relieving spasm and redistributing flow from epicardial to endocardial regions by opening up collateral channels.

Side effects include flushing, headaches and hypotension. Nitrates should not be used in patients who have hypotensive, hypertrophic obstructive cardiomyopathy.

Opioids

Indications:

Analgesia

Acute left ventricular failure (LVF)

Adult doses of 2.5–10 mg diamorphine and 5–20 mg morphine are equipotent.

Morphine and diamorphine are opioid analgesics. They reduce

both ventricular preload by increasing venous capacitance and ventricular afterload by mild arterial vasodilatation; hence they reduce myocardial oxygen demands. They may cause profound hypotension especially in the hypovolaemic patient.

Opioids should be given by IV injection and the dose titrated in 0.5–1.0 mg boluses, according to the patient's pain. This should prevent the sudden onset of profound respiratory depression, hypotension and bradycardia associated with rapid administration of larger doses. The final dose will also depend on the age and size of the patient.

Respiratory depression for hypotension can be reversed by naloxone, as described earlier. Anti-emetic drugs should be given to suppress opiate induced nausea/vomiting. Metoclopramide (10 mg IV) is probably the drug of choice. Cyclizine and prochlorperazine should not be administered as they may cause vasoconstriction and hypotension, respectively. Furthermore, the latter is not licensed for administration via this route.

Sodium bicarbonate

Indications:

Severe metabolic acidosis

Small doses of 50 mmol (50 ml 8.4%) sodium bicarbonate are given and repeated as required guided by regular blood gas monitoring.

Cardiac arrest results in combined respiratory and metabolic acidosis due to cessation of pulmonary gaseous exchange and anaerobic cellular metabolism, respectively (see Chapter 4). The most effective treatment is effective ventilation. If, however, the pH is <7.0–7.1 during or immediately following resuscitation from cardiac arrest, small doses of sodium bicarbonate may be given.

The administration of bicarbonate results in the generation of carbon dioxide, which diffuses rapidly into cells. This not only exacerbates intracellular acidosis but also has a negative inotropic effect on ischaemic myocardium. Moreover, it may present a high, osmotically active sodium load to an already compromised circulation and brain as well as producing a left shift in the oxygen dissociation curve and further inhibiting release of oxygen to the tissues.

A mild acidosis causes vasodilatation and possibly increased cerebral blood flow. Therefore, full correlation of the pH could diminish the cerebral blood flow at a particularly critical time. The bicarbonate ion is ultimately excreted as carbon dioxide via the lungs so ventilation must be increased correspondingly. A metabolic acidosis must be severe (i.e. base excess more than −10) to warrant sodium bicarbonate administration.

Thrombolytic therapy

Indications:

Myocardial infarction

Myocardial salvage/reduction of infarct size

1. Streptokinase
2. Alteplase (r-TPA)
3. Anistreplase (APSAC – anisolyated streptokinase activated complex).

Thrombolytic therapy is the only available treatment that directly influences the outcome of MI by reducing the size of the infarct. The sooner it is used from the onset of chest pain (0–6 h) the better the results, although some benefit is still obtained up to 24 h later (see Chapter 2). Myocardial salvage is possible providing thrombolytic therapy is given within 60 min; after this time, the improvement in healing and reduction in infarct size are lower. The therapy is more effective when used in combination with aspirin, 150 mg daily. Thrombolytic therapy should be given to everyone with strong evidence of MI, providing none of the specific contraindications are present.

Contraindications

1. Active internal bleeding, recent haemorrhage or a concurrent bleeding disorder.
2. Trauma or recent invasive procedures.
3. Coma, where intracranial haemorrhage cannot be excluded.
4. Potential for emboli to be thrown off as intramural thrombus is thrombolysed.
5. Profound hypotension (for streptokinase and anistreplase but not for r-TPA).
6. Suspected aortic dissection.
7. Prolonged or traumatic CPR.
8. Pregnancy.

A recent streptococcal infection is a relative contraindication to streptokinase/APSAC.

Possible consequences of the use of thrombolytic agents are bleeding or allergy. Streptokinase and anistreplase are the two agents most likely to provoke an allergic reaction, and so prophylactic IV hydrocortisone and antihistamines are given. Reperfusion arrhythmias are common with both agents.

Although streptokinase may not be as effective as the other thrombolytic agents, cost consideration ensures that it is currently the drug of choice. In the presence of a streptococcal infection or previous streptokinase infusion (>5 day; <1 year) r-TPA is the drug of choice because it is non antigenic, and rarely causes hypotension. Furthermore, conventional doses of r-TPA have been given more rapidly than usual. This is referred to as 'accelerated' or 'front-loaded' r-TPA. This regimen is reserved, by most clinicians, for patients who have a low risk of stroke and present within 3 h of symptom onset.

Verapamil

Indications:

Supraventricular tachycardia (SVT)

Angina

The dose is 5–10 mg when given IV. It should be diluted to 1 mg/ml with saline and given slowly, to a monitored patient.

Verapamil, a class IV anti-arrhythmic agent, blocks calcium channels resulting in coronary artery and peripheral vasodilatation and reduces conduction through the A-V node. Verapamil has a significant negative inotropic effect and should not be given to a patient with broad complex tachycardia of ventricular origin.

Drug interactions with digoxin and beta-blockers are most pronounced in association with IV verapamil. It interacts with digoxin, causing plasma digoxin concentrations to rise. Both drugs have a negative effect on A–V nodal conduction which may precipitate asystole.

Although oral administration of verapamil and a beta-blocker is highly effective in the treatment of both hypertension and angina, caution is required. Intravenous administration of these drugs may produce complete heart block, asystole or severe refractory hypotension. This may also develop if verapamil is used in combination with any other anti-arrhythmic agent which also has a negative inotropic effect.

Side effects in common with other vasodilators include flushing, headaches and hypotension. The hypotensive effects last for only 5–10 min, but they can be dramatic: anti-arrhythmic effects persist for about 6 h after an IV dose.

PAEDIATRIC DOSES

Adrenaline: 10–100 μg/kg IV or intraosseous.

Adenosine: 25 μg/kg as an IV stat dose, followed every 2 min by 50 μg/kg increments until success has been achieved or a maximum dose of 500 μg/kg has been given.

Amiodarone: 5 mg/kg IV over 30 min, followed by 625 μg/kg per h.

Atropine: 20 μg/kg IV or intraosseous (minimum 100 μg).

Bretylium: 5 mg/kg IV stat dose followed by 1–2 mg/kg per h.

Beta-blockers: Propranolol: 10–50 μg/kg very slowly IV, for tachy-arrhythmias if pacing is not available.

Calcium: 0.1 ml/kg of 10% calcium chloride (0.68 mmol/ml) or 0.2 ml/kg of 10% calcium gluconate (0.225 mmol/ml).

Digoxin: 10 μg/kg in three divided doses in the first 24 h. Maintenance dose is 4 μg/kg.

Dopamine/dobutamine: 1–20 μg/kg per min.

Frusemide: 1 mg/kg IV.

Isoprenaline: 0.05–0.5 μg/kg per min IV.

Lignocaine: 1 mg/kg IV.

Opiates: Diamorphine: 0.05 mg/kg; morphine: 0.1 mg/kg.

Naloxone: 0.01–0.04 mg/kg.

Sodium bicarbonate: 1 mmol/kg.

Verapamil: The normally increased sensitivity of a child's S-A and A-V nodes mean that there is a small but significant risk of inducing asystole by using verapamil. Consequently it is safer to keep vera-pamil as second or third-line treatment for SVT in children.

SUMMARY

Drugs are very important in the management of myocardial infarction, cardiac arrest and rhythm abnormalities. Therefore knowledge of indications for use, actions and side effects will facilitate the management of these conditions. However do not forget that drugs that treat arrhythmias can cause arrhythmias.

REFERENCES

ISIS-2: Randomised trial of intravenous streptokinase, oral aspirin, both, or neither among 17,187 cases of suspected acute myocardial infarction: ISIS-2. ISIS-2 (Second International Study of Infarct Survival) Collaborative Group. *Lancet.* Aug 13 1988; **2**:(8607) 349–360.

4

Acid-base balance and blood gas analysis

Objectives

After reading this chapter you should be able to:

- Understand the meanings of the commonly used terms in acid–base balance

- Understand how the body removes carbon dioxide and acid

- Understand why acidosis occurs following cardio-pulmonary arrest

- Understand why arterial and central venous bloods need to be taken following a cardiopulmonary arrest

- Understand the system for interpreting a blood gas result

- Understand how acidosis should be managed during and after cardiopulmonary arrest

- Understand how a blood sample should be taken to minimize the chances of artefactual errors

TERMINOLOGY

It is important to be clear what is meant by the terms commonly used when discussing acid–base balance.

Acids and bases

Originally the word 'acid' was used to describe the sour taste of unripe fruit but subsequently many different meanings have been attributed to it. This led to considerable confusion and misunderstanding which was not resolved until 1923, when the following definition was proposed:

An acid is any substance which is capable of providing hydrogen ions (H+)

A strong acid is a substance which will readily provide many hydrogen ions and, conversely, a weak acid provides only a few. In the body we are mainly dealing with weak acids such as carbonic acid and lactic acid.

The opposite of an acid is a base, and this is defined as any substance which 'accepts' hydrogen ions. One of the most common bases found in the body is bicarbonate (HCO_3^-).

The pH scale, acidosis, and alkalosis

The concentration of hydrogen ions in solution is usually very small, even with strong acids. This is particularly true when dealing with the acids found in the body where the hydrogen ion concentrations are in the order of 40 nanomoles/litre (nmole/l).

1 NANOMOLE = 1 BILLIONTH OF A MOLE

To gain a perspective on how tiny this is, it is interesting to compare it with the concentration of other commonly measured electrolytes. For example the plasma concentration of sodium is around 135 mmol/l i.e. 3 million times greater!

Dealing with such very small numbers is obviously difficult and so in 1909 the pH scale was developed. This scale has the advantage of being able to express any hydrogen ion concentration as a number between 1 and 14. The pH of a normal arterial blood sample lies between 7.36 and 7.44 and is equivalent to a hydrogen ion concentration of 44–36 nmole/litre.

It is important to realize that when using the pH scale, the numerical value **increases** as the concentration of hydrogen ions **decreases** (Figure 4.1). This is a consequence of the mathematical process which was used to develop the scale. Therefore an arterial blood pH below 7.36 indicates that the concentration of hydrogen ions has increased from normal. This condition is called an **acidosis**. Conversely, a pH above 7.44 would result from a reduction in the concentration of hydrogen ions. This condition is called an **alkalosis**.

Another important consequence of the derivation of the pH scale is the fact that **small changes in pH mean relatively large changes in hydrogen ion concentration**. For example, a fall in the pH from 7.40 to 7.10 means the hydrogen ion concentration has risen from 40 to 80 nmole/l i.e. it has doubled.

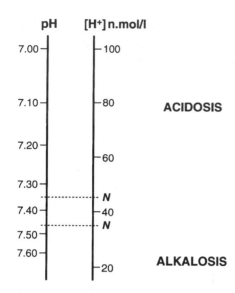

Figure 4.1   pH: Hydrogen ion scale

Summary so far

- Hydrogen ions are present in the body only in very low concentrations
- As the hydrogen ion concentration increases the pH falls
- As the hydrogen ion concentration falls the pH rises
- An acidosis occurs when the pH falls below 7.36 and an alkalosis when it rises above 7.44
- Small changes in the pH scale represent large changes in the concentration of hydrogen ions

Buffers

Many of the complex chemical reactions occurring at a cellular level are controlled by special proteins called enzymes. These substances can function effectively only at very narrow ranges of pH (7.36–7.44). However, during normal activity the body produces massive amounts of hydrogen ions which, if left unchecked, would lead to significant falls in pH. Clearly a system is required to prevent these hydrogen ions causing large changes in pH before they are eliminated from the body. This is achieved by the 'buffers' which 'take up' the free hydrogen ions in the cells and the bloodstream, thereby preventing a change in pH.

There are a variety of buffers in the body. Intracellularly the main ones are proteins, phosphate and haemoglobin. Extracellularly there are also plasma proteins and bicarbonate. Proteins 'soak-up' the hydrogen ions like a sponge and transport them to their place of elimination from the body. In the majority of cases this is at the kidneys. In contrast, the bicarbonate reacts with the hydrogen ions to produce water and carbon dioxide:

$$H^+ + HCO_3^- \rightleftharpoons H_2O + CO_2$$

The carbon dioxide is subsequently removed by the lungs.

With these common terms defined, let us now consider why people can become acidotic and how the body tries to correct it.

ACID PRODUCTION AND ITS REMOVAL

All of us, whether we are healthy or ill, produce large amounts of water, acid and carbon dioxide each day – indeed, a healthy adult will normally produce 14 570 000 000 nmole of hydrogen ions each day as part of the waste products of food metabolized to release energy. As this process occurs at a cellular level it is here that these products initially accumulate. Irreparable cellular damage would result if this was left unchecked.

The first acute compensatory mechanism is the intracellular buffering system. As described previously, this provides the cell with a temporary way of minimizing the fluctuations in acidity. Subsequently these waste products (carbon dioxide and hydrogen ions) are excreted into the bloodstream where they are taken up by the extracellular buffers (Figure 4.2).

However, this is only a temporary solution because there is only a limited amount of buffer in the body. If this was the sum total of the body's defence to acids and carbon dioxide then the buffers would soon be exhausted and the products of metabolism would accumulate in the bloodstream. A system is therefore needed to remove these harmful substances so that they do not reach toxic levels and, at the same time, regenerate the buffers. Fortunately the body can eliminate these waste products by the lungs and the kidneys.

**Figure 4.2
Removal of
waste products
from cells**

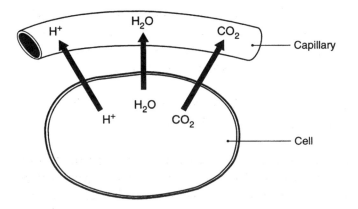

Carbon dioxide removal (the respiratory component)

Carbon dioxide (CO_2) released from cells is transported in the blood to the lungs, diffuses into the alveoli, and is ultimately removed from the body during expiration (Figure 4.3).

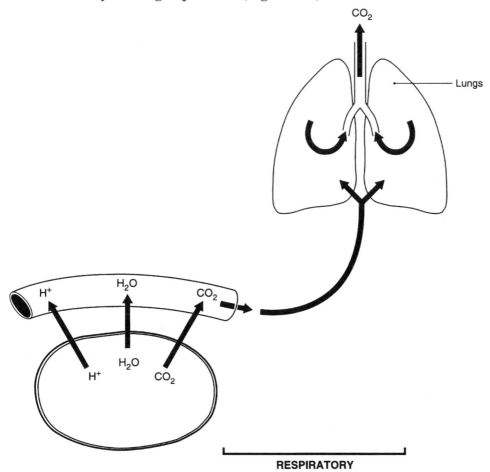

**Figure 4.3
Removal of CO_2
by the lungs**

If CO_2 is produced faster than it can be eliminated, or there is a blockage to its elimination, then it will accumulate in the blood-stream. Here it reacts with water in the plasma with the result that hydrogen ions (H^+) are produced along with bicarbonate:

$$CO_2 + H_2O \rightleftharpoons H^+ + HCO_3^-$$

The greater the amount of CO_2, the more H^+ produced. If this causes the pH to fall below 7.36 then an **acidosis** has been produced. As the cause of the acidosis in this case is the problem in the respiratory system, it is known as a **respiratory acidosis**.

If a sample of arterial blood was taken immediately this occurred then the result shown in Table 4.1 would be obtained.

As a byproduct of the reaction between carbon dioxide and water, the bicarbonate concentration also increases by the same amount as the hydrogen ions. However, this increase is usually very small.

41

Table 4.1

	Normal	Respiratory acidosis
pH	7.36–7.44	↓↓
$Paco_2$	36–40 mmHg, 4.8–5.3 kPa	↑↑↑
HCO_3^-	21–27 (mmol/l)	↑

Consequently these changes in concentration are enough to change the pH scale but are not large enough to alter significantly the plasma bicarbonate concentration.

In a normal person at rest the respiratory component will excrete at least 13 000 000 000 nanomoles of H^+ per day. It is therefore easy to see that there can be a rapid onset of acidosis during episodes of hypoventilation.

Acid removal (the metabolic component)

As has already been described, acids are continually produced as a result of cellular metabolism. The amount produced from normal metabolism is approximately 1 570 000 000 nmole/day. This acid load is soaked up by buffers in the bloodstream and transported safely to their point of elimination (Figure 4.4).

One of the buffers is bicarbonate (HCO_3^-). This is generated by the kidneys and released into the bloodstream where it reacts with free hydrogen (Figure 4.5).

In certain circumstances so much acid is produced by the cells that it exceeds the capacity of both the protein buffers and bicarbonate. If this causes the pH to fall below 7.36 then an acidosis has been produced. As this is a result of a defect in the metabolic system, it is termed a **metabolic acidosis**.

If a sample of arterial blood is taken when this occurs the result shown in Table 4.2 would be obtained:

Table 4.2

	Normal	Metabolic acidosis
pH	7.36–7.44	↓↓
$Paco_2$	36–40 mmHg, 4.8–5.3 kPa	36–40 mmHg, 4.8–5.3 kPa
HCO_3^-	21–27 (mmol/l)	↓

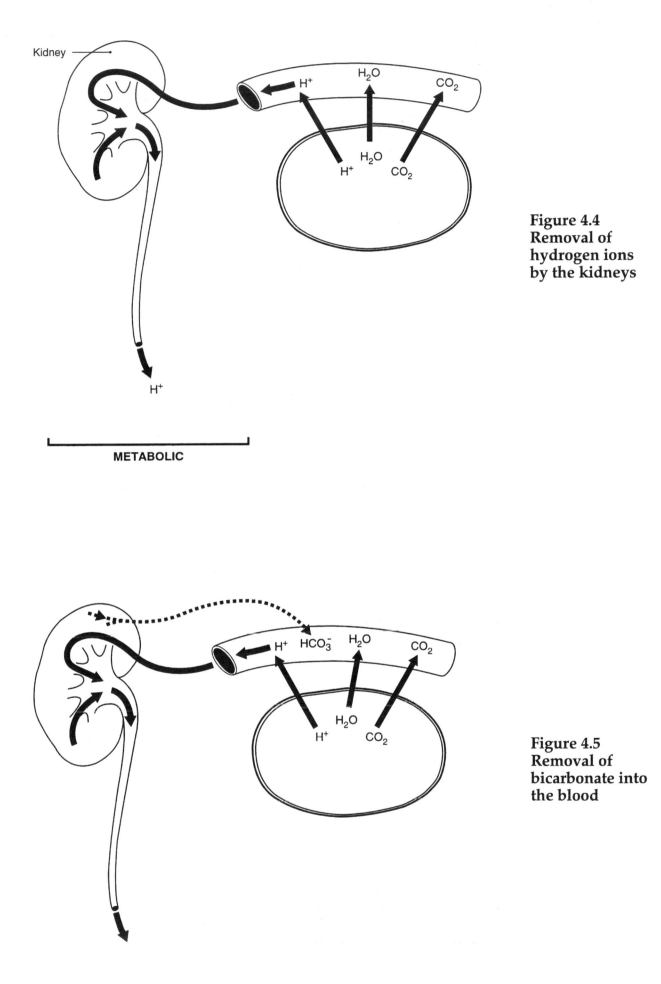

Figure 4.4
Removal of
hydrogen ions
by the kidneys

METABOLIC

Figure 4.5
Removal of
bicarbonate into
the blood

The bicarbonate level has fallen as a consequence of reacting with the free hydrogen ions to produce carbon dioxide and water.

Summary so far

- Carbon dioxide and acids are being produced continually by cellular metabolism
- The removal of CO_2 by the lungs is termed the respiratory component
- The removal of acid by the kidneys is termed the metabolic component

The respiratory-metabolic link

It can be seen from the above that the body has two distinct methods of preventing the accumulation of hydrogen ions and the subsequent development of an acidosis. As a further protection against acidosis these two components are in balance (or equilibrium) so that each can **compensate** for a derangement in the other.

This link between the respiratory and metabolic systems is due to the presence of **carbonic acid** (H_2CO_3) (Figure 4.6).

This ability of each system to compensate for the other becomes more marked when the initial disturbance in one system is prolonged.

The production of carbonic acid is dependant upon an enzyme called carbonic anhydrase which is present in abundance in the red cells and the kidneys. It is therefore ideally placed to facilitate the link between the respiratory and the metabolic systems.

Let us consider how this link can help the body respond to an excess of either carbon dioxide or acid.

Example 1

In a patient with inadequate alveolar ventilation, e.g. chronic bronchitis, carbon dioxide accumulates. As we have seen, this will tend to cause a respiratory acidosis. Rather than the body existing in a chronic state of acidosis, the metabolic system can help to compensate by increasing bicarbonate production by the kidneys. Utilizing the carbonic acid link this enables the removal of some of the excess carbon dioxide (Figure 4.7) – i.e. the metabolic system is compensating for the respiratory system. However, this takes several days to

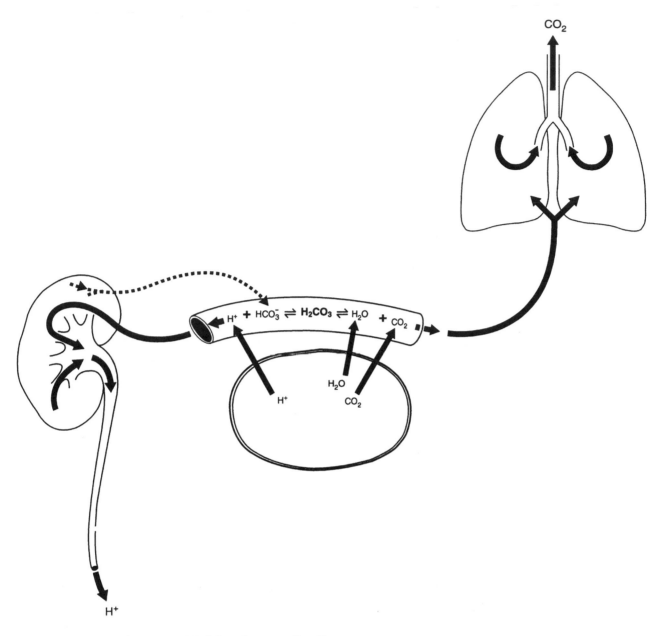

$$H^+ + HCO_3^- \rightleftharpoons H_2CO_3 \rightleftharpoons H_2O + CO_2$$

Figure 4.6   Carbonic acid–bicarbonate buffer

become effective as it is dependant upon the increased production of enzymes in the kidney.

It is important to realize that in the acute situation **the body never over-compensates**. An arterial blood sample taken at this time will demonstrate that there is still a persistent but slight underlying acidosis (Table 4.3).

Example 2

Diabetic patients sometimes develop a state of excess acid production known as **diabetic ketoacidosis**. The excess cellular acid is

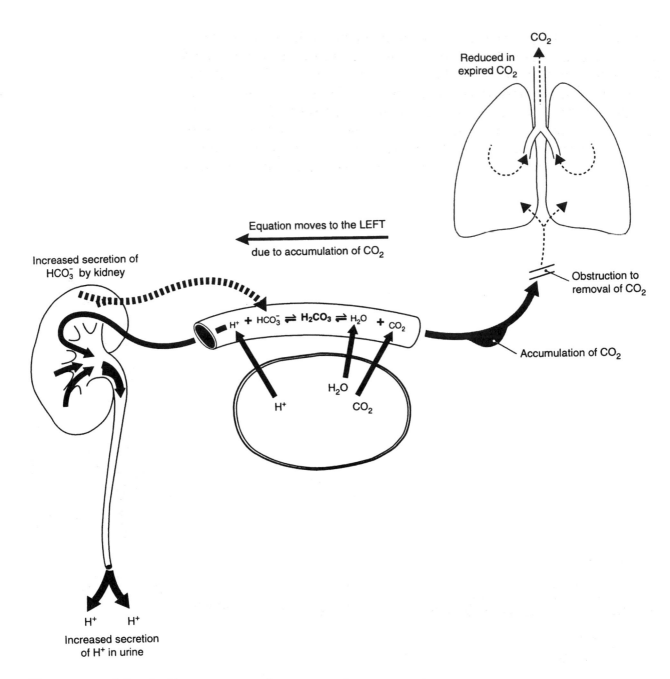

Figure 4.7 Metabolic compensation to respiratory acidosis

Table 4.3

	Normal	Respiratory acidosis	Metabolic compensation
pH	7.36–7.44	↓↓	↓
Pa_{CO_2}	36–40 mmHg, 4.8–5.3 kPa	↑	↑
HCO_3^-	21–27 mmol/l	↑	↑↑

released into the plasma to be transported to the kidney for excretion. However, the kidneys are able to excrete the additional acid load only slowly and a metabolic acidosis develops. The kidneys are slowly stimulated into increasing bicarbonate production to counteract this but it takes several days. In the meantime, because of the carbonic acid link, some of the excess acid can be converted to carbon dioxide and eliminated by the respiratory system (Figure 4.8) – i.e. the respiratory system has compensated for the metabolic system.

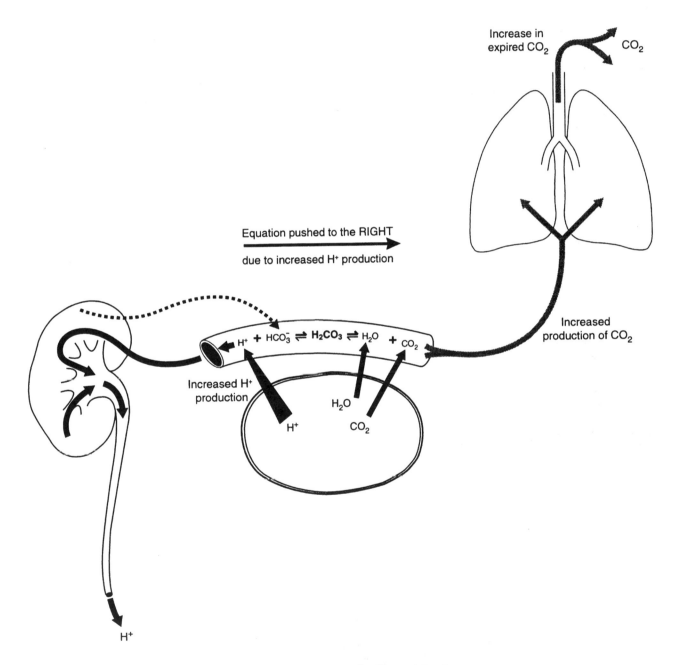

Equation pushed to the RIGHT due to increased H$^+$ production

$$H^+ + HCO_3^- \rightleftharpoons H_2CO_3 \rightleftharpoons H_2O + CO_2$$

Increased H$^+$ production

H$^+$

H$_2$O

CO$_2$

Increased production of CO$_2$

Increase in expired CO$_2$

CO$_2$

H$^+$

Figure 4.8 Respiratory compensation to metabolic acidosis

This compensation is facilitated by the fact that the excess hydrogen ions are detected by special receptors in the brain which, in turn, increase the respiratory rate and depth within minutes (compare this with the slow response of the kidneys). This process enables the body to eliminate the extra carbon dioxide, providing there is no obstruction to ventilation. The lowering of the carbon dioxide levels in the blood encourages further free acid to be converted into carbonic acid and eventually carbon dioxide.

However, the body **never over-compensates in the acute situation**. Therefore, even after several hours, respiratory compensation will only be partial and the blood will still be slightly acidotic (Table 4.4).

Table 4.4

	Normal	Metabolic acidosis	Respiratory compensation
pH	7.36–7.44	$\downarrow\downarrow$	$\downarrow$
Pa_{CO_2}	36–40 mmHg, 4.8–5.3 kPa	36–40 mmHg, 4.8–5.3 kPa	$\downarrow$
HCO_3^-	21–27 mmol/l	$\downarrow$	$\downarrow$

It must also be remembered that the degree to which the respiratory system can compensate is dependant upon the work involved in breathing and the systemic effects of a low arterial concentration of carbon dioxide.

Summary so far

- The metabolic component of the body's acid elimination mechanism can compensate for a respiratory acidosis by increasing the production of bicarbonate by the kidneys

- Compensation by the metabolic component usually takes days to achieve

- The respiratory component of the body's acid elimination mechanism can compensate for a metabolic acidosis by increasing ventilation of the lungs and eliminating carbon dioxide

- Compensation by the respiratory component usually takes place within minutes

- In the acute situation the body never over-compensates; therefore the underlying acidosis will remain

Combined metabolic and respiratory acidosis

It follows from the above description that should both the metabolic and respiratory systems be defective, or inadequate to the body's needs, then the accumulation of acid and carbon dioxide will be unchecked. An example of this particularly dire situation is seen in patients suffering from a cardiorespiratory arrest. As a result cells of the body produce lactic acid because they are being starved of oxygen. In addition, carbon dioxide accumulates in the cells and blood because it can no longer be excreted by the lungs due to the failure of ventilation (Figure 4.9).

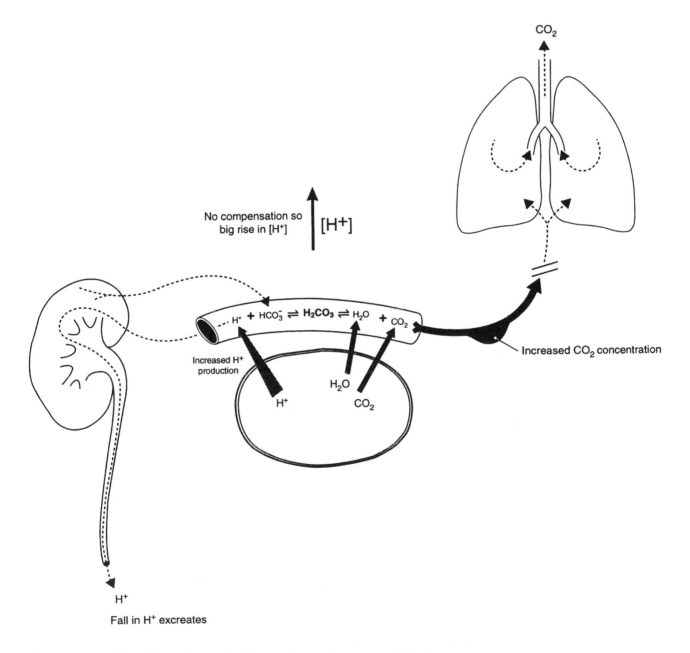

Figure 4.9   Combined metabolic and respiratory acidosis

An arterial blood sample taken at this time would therefore demonstrate a combined respiratory and metabolic acidosis (Table 4.5).

Table 4.5

	Normal	Respiratory and metabolic acidosis
pH	7.36–7.44	↓↓↓↓
$Pa\text{co}_2$	36–40 mmHg, 4.8–5.3 kPa	↑↑
HCO_3^-	21–27 mmol/l	↓↓

CENTRAL VENOUS AND ARTERIAL BLOOD SAMPLES

So far we have concentrated on arterial blood sampling and analysis. This is blood which has had the benefit of passing through the lungs, where carbon dioxide can be eliminated and oxygen taken up. In contrast, central venous blood (blood in the right atrium) is a mixture of all the blood returning to the heart from the body's tissues. It therefore has a high concentration of the body's waste products and low levels of oxygen (Table 4.6).

Table 4.6

	Arterial	Central venous
pH	7.36–7.44	7.31–7.40
$Pa\text{co}_2$	36–40 mmHg, 4.8–5.3 kPa	41–51 mmHg, 5.5–6.8 kPa
HCO_3^-	21–27 mmol/l	25–29 mmol/l
$P\text{o}_2$ on air	>80 mmHg, >10.6 kPa	38–42 mmHg, 5.1–5.6 kPa

Compare this with what occurs during a cardiorespiratory arrest. In the absence of cardiopulmonary resuscitation no blood will go through ventilated lungs. Therefore the arterial sample and central venous sample will be **approximately the same.**

In contrast, following endotracheal intubation, artificial ventilation and external chest compression, the carbon dioxide delivered to the alveoli is easily cleared by mechanical ventilation and some oxygen is taken up. Indeed, removal of carbon dioxide can be so effective that there is a marked reduction in $Pa\text{co}_2$ and a paradoxical respiratory alkalosis (low arterial carbon dioxide concentration despite high venous carbon dioxide and acidosis) develops. Consequently, the arterial pH can be neutral, mildly acidotic or even alkalotic depending upon how much carbon dioxide is being removed. Severe arterial acidosis in a patient receiving cardiopulmonary resuscitation indicates that resuscitation is inadequate, i.e. there is inadequate blood flow to the lungs or inadequate ventilation either separately or as a combination of both together.

The arterial sample taken during the resuscitation of a patient with a cardiorespiratory arrest is simply demonstrating the clinician's ability to remove carbon dioxide and add oxygen. The patient's true 'acid' state (pH, carbon dioxide and bicarbonate levels) is more accurately deduced from analysis of blood from a central vein.

A SYSTEMATIC APPROACH FOR ANALYSING A BLOOD GAS SAMPLE

There are many similarities between analysing a blood gas result and interpreting a rhythm strip. In both cases it is important to assess the patient first and to be aware of the clinical history and current medications. A review of the other laboratory investigations is also helpful. In the emergency situation, however, these data may not be immediately available and you will have to interpret the initial results with caution and follow trends whilst the rest of the information is being obtained.

The system

There are several systems for interpreting blood gas results in the emergency situation. The one described below is an effective system based upon a series of questions (Box 4.1).

Box 4.1   Questions used in interpreting a blood gas sample

- Is the patient acidotic or alkalotic?
- Is the abnormality due to a defect in the respiratory system?
- Is the abnormality due to a defect in the metabolic system?
- Is there compensation or a combined respiratory and metabolic defect?
- Is the patient hypoxic?

Is the patient acidotic or alkalotic?

As the body does not over-compensate in the acute situation, determining the acid/alkali state of the patient will enable you to detect the primary problem – i.e. has the patient got too much acid or too much alkali? The question can be answered by checking the pH. An acidosis is present when the pH is less than 7.36 and an alkalosis when it is over 7.44.

Is the abnormality due to a defect in the respiratory component?

Checking the Pa_{CO_2} gives a good indication of the ventilatory adequacy because it is inversely proportional to alveolar ventilation. When combined with pH measurement it can be used to determine if there is either, a problem with the respiratory system, or if the respiratory component is simply compensating for a problem in the metabolic component.

Take for example an arterial sample with a pH of 7.2 and a Pa_{CO_2} of 60 mmHg (8.0 kPa). A pH of 7.2 indicates that there is an acidosis and as the Pa_{CO_2} is raised this indicates that there is a respiratory acidosis. Consider now a patient with a similar pH but a Pa_{CO_2} of 25 mmHg (3.3 kPa). There is still an acidosis but the lowered Pa_{CO_2} would imply there is respiratory compensation to a metabolic acidosis. To confirm this the metabolic component would need to be assessed (see below).

Is the abnormality due to a defect in the metabolic component?

To determine the metabolic component, the concentration of bicarbonate is measured. In a similar situation to that described above, when the bicarbonate concentration is combined with pH one can determine if there is either a primary metabolic or compensatory metabolic problem.

Using the example above, the bicarbonate was found to be 9.5 mmol/l. This is below the normal range (22–27 mmol/l). A pH of 7.2 and a Pa_{CO_2} of 25 mmHg (3.3 kPa) is in keeping with the idea that this patient has a respiratory compensation to a metabolic acidosis.

It is important to realize that not all laboratories measure bicarbonate: instead the base deficit is calculated. This is defined as the number of moles of **bicarbonate** which must be added to the equivalent of 1 litre of the patient's blood so that a pH of 7.4 is produced. Respiratory influences are eliminated by keeping the partial pressure of carbon dioxide constant at 40 mmHg (5.3 kPa). The value should be zero but a normal range is –2 to +2 mmol/l.

For example, an arterial blood sample with a pH of 7.25, a $Paco_2$ of 25 mmHg (3.3 kPa) and a base deficit of –15 indicates there is a metabolic acidosis with a compensatory respiratory alkalosis.

The base deficit is used to help calculate the dose of bicarbonate which should be given to a patient to correct the metabolic acidosis. However, it is important to realize that a slight metabolic acidosis is beneficial because it facilitates the release of oxygen from the haemoglobin molecule to the tissues. Consequently a deficit is only treated if it is large, i.e. more negative than –6.

Is there compensation or a combined respiratory and metabolic defect?

Ideally a defect in either the respiratory or the metabolic system is compensated by changes in the other system. It is therefore important to ascertain that this is the case and that the abnormality is not due to a combined metabolic and respiratory acidosis. For example an arterial blood sample with a pH of 7.1, with a $Paco_2$ of 50 mmHg (6.7 kPa) and a base deficit of –15 indicates there is a combined acidosis.

Is the patient hypoxic?

The partial pressure of oxygen in an arterial sample must be interpreted in the light of the inspired concentration of oxygen (Fio_2). Since atmospheric pressure is approximately 100 kPa, 1% is about 1 kPa (7.5 mmHg). This would mean inspiring 30% oxygen from a facemask would lead to an **arterial concentration** of around 20–25 kPa (150–187.5 mmHg). This apparent fall is due to the normal drop of about 7.5 kPa (56 mmHg) between the partial pressure of oxygen inspired at the mouth and that in the alveoli. A drop significantly greater than 10 kPa (75 mmHg) would imply there is a mismatch in the lungs between ventilation and perfusion with blood.

Example

Using this system for interpreting blood gases let us now consider the following case.

A 17-year-old schoolgirl is found at home by her parents in a restless and confused state. She is pale, sweaty and hyperventilating. The arterial blood gases and electrolytes, while breathing room air, are:

pH   7.10
$Paco_2$ 18 mmHg (2.4 kPa)
Base deficit   –14
Po_2 105 mmHg (14 kPa)

Is the patient acidotic or alkalotic?
The pH is 7.1 which is below 7.36. Therefore there is an acidosis.

Is the abnormality due to a defect in the respiratory system?
The $Pa\text{CO}_2$ is low. This implies that the respiratory system is compensating for a metabolic acidosis. It is therefore unlikely that there is a defect in the respiratory system.

Is the abnormality due to a defect in the metabolic system?
The base deficit is very low, indicating there is a metabolic acidosis, i.e. a defect in the metabolic system.

Is there compensation or a combined respiratory and metabolic defect?
There is respiratory compensation for the metabolic acidosis as already described.

Is the patient hypoxic?
There is no evidence of hypoxia or a ventilatory-perfusion mismatch in the lungs.

As there are many causes for a metabolic acidosis, you will now need to carry out further investigations. A common initial test is to determine the patient's **anion gap**. This is defined as the difference in concentration between the cation (i.e. sodium and potassium) and the anions (i.e. bicarbonate and chloride). It is due to the presence of unmeasured anions such as phosphate, sulphate and albumin and is normally between 8 and 16 mmole/l.

The causes of metabolic acidosis can be divided into those associated with and without an increased gap. The latter is by far the most common and the causes giving rise to this can be remembered using the mnemonic **MUDSLEEP** (Table 4.7).

Table 4.7   Causes of metabolic acidosis

Anion gap less than 16 mmol/l	Anion gap greater than 16 mmol/l
Renal tubular acidosis	Methanol toxicity
Acetazolamide overdose	Uraemia
Bicarbonate loss from the gut	Diabetic ketoacidosis
	Salicylate overdose
	Lactic acidosis
	Ethanol overdose
	Ethylene glycol toxicity
	Paraldehyde overdose

The patient's blood sample can now be analysed further by measuring the appropriate electrolyte concentrations. In this case these were found to be:

Na^+ 135 mmol/l
K^+ 5.0 mmol/l
HCO_3 10 mmol/l
Chloride   95 mmol/l

Using this information it is possible to determine the anion gap:

Anion gap = (sodium + potassium) – (bicarbonate + chloride)
= (135 + 5) – (10 + 95)
= 35 mmole/l

The most likely cause of a metabolic acidosis with an increased anion gap in a previously healthy adolescent is an overdose or diabetic ketoacidosis. Consequently the salicylate and blood sugar levels must be checked in this patient.

MANAGEMENT OF ACIDOSIS DUE TO A CARDIOPULMONARY ARREST

The respiratory and metabolic acidosis which results from a cardiopulmonary arrest should initially be managed by effective CPR and hyperventilation with 100% oxygen. These provide the most effective way of eliminating the carbon dioxide and reducing the production of lactic acid by increasing the body's uptake of oxygen.

Bicarbonate is not the treatment of choice to correct the acidosis because it reacts with the hydrogen ions and increases local carbon dioxide production. Unless there is adequate ventilation this will rapidly diffuse into cells and increases the intracellular acidosis. Hypernatraemia and hyperosmolar states are also common following sodium bicarbonate administration. Furthermore the arterial alkalosis, produced by injection of bicarbonate, leads to a left shift of the oxyhaemoglobin dissociation curve and a reduction in the oxygen delivery to the tissues. Indeed, for each 0.1 rise in pH there is a drop of around 10% in the tissue oxygen availability.

The disparity between the level of acidosis measured in a central venous sample and that in an arterial sample becomes marked when there is prolonged resuscitation (over 10 minutes) or following restoration of the cardiopulmonary arrest. In the latter case considerable quantities of lactic acid are 'washed out' of the peripheral tissues by the restored blood supply and carried to the central veins.

In these situations small doses of bicarbonate may occasionally be used. Nevertheless, increased ventilation will still be required to excrete the excess carbon dioxide generated.

As 1 mmole of bicarbonate equals 1 ml of 8.4% bicarbonate, the amount required is also the number of millilitres of 8.4% solution. In practice, however, smaller doses, either one-third of that calculated or 50 mmole (50 ml of 8.4% bicarbonate), are given and the effect monitored preferably by repeat analysis of a central venous sample or, if not available, an arterial sample.

SUMMARY

The body's system for removing the carbon dioxide and acid produced by metabolism has both a respiratory and metabolic component. These are linked by carbonic acid which enables one component to compensate for a defect in the other. In cardiopulmonary arrest both components are defective. Consequently there is no compensation and the pH falls markedly. This must be managed with effective cardiopulmonary resuscitation and adequate ventilation. Only when both these treatments have been introduced should the administration of bicarbonate be contemplated.

SECTION TWO
Life support

—— 5 ——
Basic life support

Objectives

After reading this chapter you should be able to:

- Understand the reason for basic life support
- Describe the SAFE approach to a patient
- Evaluate the condition of a collapsed patient
- Understand the methods used to provide support of the airway, breathing and circulation
- Place a collapsed patient in the recovery position
- Understand the methods used to deal with a choking patient

Basic life support skills are always a pre-requisite to learning advanced cardiac life support skills, in both children and adults

INTRODUCTION

Collapsed patients require assistance to maintain their airway, breathing and circulation in order to prevent further deterioration in their condition. When this is achieved without the use of any equipment, it is termed **basic life support** (BLS). This must be continued whilst further help is summoned to diagnose and treat the cause of the collapse.

More recently, the use of simple protective shields interposed between the mouths of the rescuer and patient, for example the Laerdal Pocket Mask, has become more widespread. This is sometimes referred to as **basic life support with airway adjunct**.

This chapter will concentrate on the principles of adult BLS. Paediatric BLS will be covered in detail in Chapter 12.

REASON FOR BASIC LIFE SUPPORT

Following a cardiorespiratory arrest ('cardiac arrest'), irreversible brain damage occurs within 3–4 min. Survival is most likely when the event is witnessed and a bystander commences resuscitation. Studies have indicated that survival is also improved when the time from collapse to initiation of BLS is short. Furthermore, it has been postulated that speed of initiation may be more important than the absolute quality of the technique employed. Therefore, in general, BLS should be started for all people who have suddenly become unresponsive **and** are either not breathing (apnoeic) or have an absent major pulse, or both. The only exception to this is if the cardiorespiratory arrest occurs in hospital and an up-to-date, signed, 'not for resuscitation' order is in force.

In order that the rescuer suffers no harm, and that BLS is carried out appropriately and in the most efficient manner, the following sequence of actions should be performed.

THE SAFE APPROACH

On discovering or being asked to attend to a collapsed patient, the first response must be to **S**hout for help. BLS is physically demanding and more effectively performed by two rescuers. Furthermore, the arrival of any help also allows earlier summoning of advanced help (see later).

Patients may collapse anywhere, at any time, from many causes. The rescuer must **A**pproach the patient with care, never putting himself (or others) at risk. This is particularly important when the collapse occurs outside hospital, where there may be toxic fumes, traffic, electricity, or fire endangering both the rescuer and patient.

If there are risks to either the victim or the rescuers, then these should be removed. The patient must be **F**ree from danger, or moved to a place of safety before starting resuscitation.

Finally, the rescuer must **E**valuate the patient's **A**irway, **B**reathing and **C**irculation (the **ABC system**). Not all collapsed patients will need or appreciate expired air (artificial) ventilation and external cardiac compressions.

On finding a collapsed patient:

Shout for help
Approach with care
Free from danger
Evaluate ABC

PATIENT EVALUATION

Assess if the patient is conscious. This is achieved by placing one hand on the patient's forehead, shaking the shoulders gently with the other hand and at the same time asking loudly: 'Are you all right?'

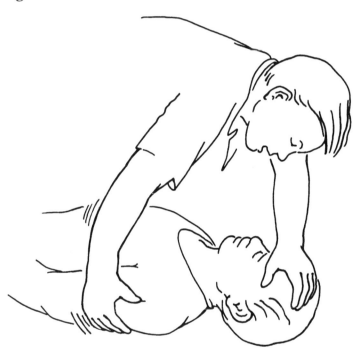

Figure 5.1 'Are you all right?'

One of two things may happen and will determine further action.

The patient responds by either talking or moving

If it is safe to do so, leave him in the position in which he was found, whilst additional help is summoned. However, remember that he may deteriorate before help arrives, so reassessment is mandatory. If this does happen, proceed as detailed below.

Points to note:

- The head is held stable during the evaluation to guard against the possibility of aggravating a cervical spine injury.
- Always assume the patient might be deaf, therefore ensure he can see your lips move.
- In the responsive patient, where there is obvious trauma, immobilize the cervical spine by in-line stabilization until help arrives (Figure 5.2).

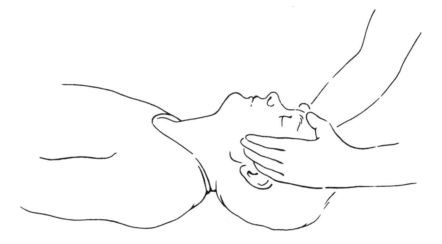

Figure 5.2 In-line stabilization

There is no response to voice or touch

Shout for help again if none has arrived and then evaluate the patient's airway, breathing and circulation, the ABC system.

THE ABCs

Airway

In most unconscious patients the airway will become obstructed. This occurs at the level of the hypopharynx as the reduced tone in the muscles of the tongue, jaw and neck allow the tongue to fall against the posterior pharyngeal wall (Figure 5.3). Airway obstruction may be the primary problem and correction of this might allow recovery without further intervention. The following manoeuvres are designed to achieve this.

Head tilt plus chin lift

The rescuer's hand nearest the head is placed on the forehead, gently tilting (extending) the head backwards. The chin is then

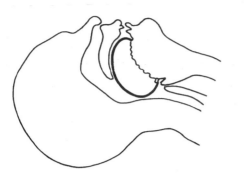

**Figure 5.3
Sagittal section
of the airway**

lifted using the index and middle finger of the rescuer's other hand. If this causes the mouth to close, it may be necessary to use the thumb to part the lips (Figure 5.4).

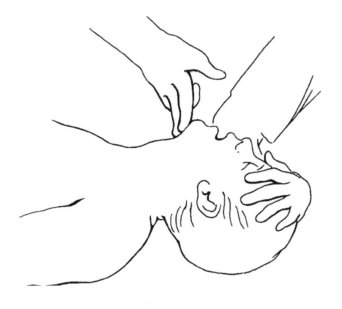

**Figure 5.4
Chin lift**

Jaw thrust

If the above technique fails to create an airway, or there is a suspicion of a cervical spine injury then the 'jaw thrust' must be used. The patient's jaw is thrust upwards (forwards) by applying pressure behind the angles of the mandible. This can be achieved by the rescuer using his thumbs or the tips of his fingers, while resting the base of the thumbs on the patient's cheeks.

As this manoeuvre is combined with a head tilt, and the tips of the thumbs are used to open the mouth, it is often referred to as the 'triple airway manoeuvre'.

Finger sweep

If there is any evidence that foreign material may be contributing to airway obstruction the mouth must be opened and inspected. Any obvious material should be removed by placing a finger in the mouth and gently sweeping from side to back 'hooking' out loose material. At the same time, broken, loose or partial dentures must be removed, but well fitting ones should be left in place (see below).

**Figure 5.5
Finger sweep**

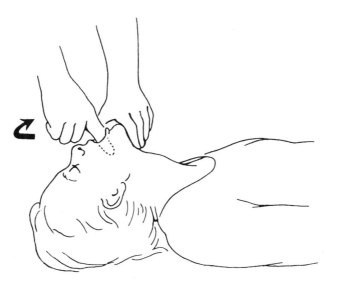

Breathing

Having created an airway using one of the above techniques, the patient's breathing must now be evaluated immediately, in the following manner:

- **Look** down the line of the chest to see if it is rising and falling.
- **Listen** at the mouth and nose for breath sounds, gurgling or snoring sounds.
- **Feel** for expired air at the patient's mouth and nose with the side of the rescuer's cheek.

Look, listen and feel for up to 10 s before deciding whether breathing is absent (Figure 5.6).

The patient is breathing (not just intermittent gasps)

Place the patient in the recovery position (see later) unless it is unsafe to do so because of other injuries. Then seek help. Once this has been achieved the patient should be kept under close supervision to ensure that his airway remains patent and breathing

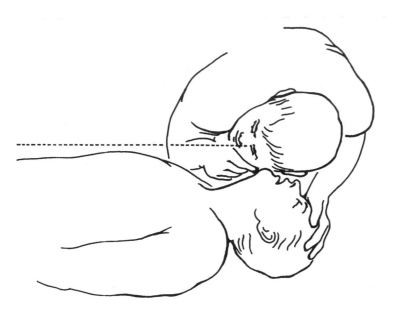

**Figure 5.6
Look, listen, feel
technique**

adequate. The circulation must also be checked if there is any change in his condition (see below).

The patient is not breathing

Help must be sought, even though for a single rescuer this may mean temporarily leaving the patient to get to a telephone. On return commence expired air ventilation immediately with two breaths of expired air, each lasting 1.5–2 s. If there is any difficulty achieving effective ventilation, remember to check the mouth for any foreign material and ensure that the head tilt and chin lift or jaw thrust are being maintained. Up to five initial attempts are allowed to achieve two ventilations of adequate volume. An assessment must now be made of the circulation.

Circulation

Look for signs of a circulation; movement or swallowing, or by feeling for a pulse. In an emergency, central arteries are more reliable than peripheral ones and the carotid artery is usually the most accessible and acceptable. The carotid artery is found on either side of the neck in the 'gutter' between the larynx and sternomastoid muscle.

It is important not to take more than 10 s before deciding that the circulation is absent.

The patient is not breathing but does have a pulse

Continue expired air ventilation, observing between breaths to see if the patient makes any attempt at spontaneous ventilation. Approximately every minute, recheck the circulation by feeling for

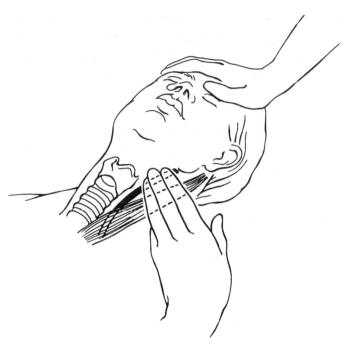

**Figure 5.7
Feeling for the
carotid pulse**

a major pulse. This should not take more than 10 s on each occasion. Should the victim start to breathe, turn him into the recovery position if safe to do so. Monitor breathing and circulation regularly as described and recommence expired air ventilation if spontaneous ventilation ceases.

The patient is not breathing and does not have a pulse

This is often referred to as a 'cardiac arrest', and it is essential that respiratory and circulatory support are provided effectively. If necessary the victim must be carefully placed in the supine position on a firm surface and resuscitation commenced.

Two expired air ventilations are followed by 15 external cardiac compressions. This cycle (2:15) should be performed continuously, remembering to tilt the head and lift the chin to create a patent airway and to check the correct position of the hands before starting cardiac compressions. If a second rescuer is available quickly decide who is to perform which function, then commence ventilation and external cardiac compression. When there are two rescuers the cycle changes to one breath followed by five compressions. This cycle (1:5) is performed continuously and each breath should last for approximately 1.5–2 s. Cardiac compression should stop momentarily to allow ventilation then recommence without waiting for exhalation. In order to minimize delays between each series of compressions and ventilation, it may be helpful for the person performing compressions to count out each compression.

The person performing external cardiac compression can leave his hands on the sternum between each series of compressions, but in order not to reduce the efficacy of ventilation, must totally release the pressure. Two-person BLS is best performed from opposite sides of the patient. This allows the rescuers to change activity with minimum disruption in case of fatigue.

This combination of expired air ventilation and external cardiac compression is frequently referred to as **cardiopulmonary resuscitation (CPR)**. Once started, it must not be interrupted unless:

- The patient shows signs of spontaneous ventilation or movement. If this does happen, then the carotid pulse should be reassessed for no more than 10 s before deciding how to continue. Unfortunately, such an occurrence is extremely rare.
- Qualified help arrives.
- You become physically exhausted.

Getting help

When faced with the problem of providing resuscitation, whatever the circumstances, you should seek help as quickly as possible. When more than one person trained in performing BLS is immediately available quickly decide who starts resuscitation and who goes for help. When there is only one person available, the dilemma arises as to whether to start resuscitation or summon help first. It is suggested that in this situation, if the patient has suffered **trauma, drowning** or is a **child** or **infant**, a single person should perform resuscitation for approximately 1 min (using paediatric protocols if appropriate) before leaving to get help. However, most adult cases are likely to be primarily cardiac problems and **help must be sought immediately you have established that they are not breathing.**

The technique of expired air ventilation

To successfully ventilate a patient with expired air there must be a clear path, with no leaks, between the rescuer's lungs and the patient's lungs.

Mouth to mouth ventilation

1. The patient's airway is kept patent by the rescuer, using the palm of his uppermost hand to perform a head tilt, leaving the index finger and thumb free to pinch the patient's nose to prevent leaks. The fingers of the lower hand are then used to perform a chin lift, and if necessary the thumb is used to open the mouth.

2. The rescuer takes a deep breath in and makes a seal with his lips around the patient's mouth. Well fitting dentures are often left in place as they help to maintain the contour of the mouth and make it easier to create a good seal.
3. The rescuer then exhales into the patient's mouth for 1.5–2 s, at the same time listening for leaks and looking down at the patient's chest to ensure it rises (in an adult this requires a volume of 400–500 ml).
4. Maintaining the head tilt/chin lift, the rescuer should then move away from the patient's mouth to allow passive exhalation for 2–4 s, watching to make sure the chest falls.

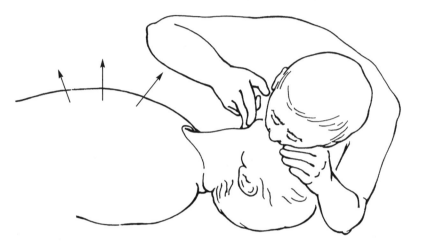

**Figure 5.8
Mouth to mouth
ventilation**

Mouth to nose ventilation

This technique is used if mouth to mouth ventilation is unsuccessful, e.g. if an obstruction in the mouth cannot be removed or if the rescuer is a child. The airway is maintained as already described, but the mouth is closed with the fingers of the lower hand. A seal is made between the rescuer's lips around the base of the patient's nose. The rescuer then exhales into the nose for 1.5–2 s, checking as described previously for successful ventilation. The patient's mouth can be opened to assist with expiration, for 2–4 s, whilst the rescuer watches to ensure that the chest falls.

Each complete cycle of expired air ventilation should take approximately 6 s, allowing 10 breaths per minute.

Common causes of inadequate ventilation

- Obstruction: Failing to maintain head tilt, chin lift.
- Leaks: Inadequate seal around the mouth or failure to occlude the patient's nose.
- Exhaling too hard: Trying to overcome an obstructed airway, resulting in gastric distension.
- Foreign body: Unrecognized in the patient's airway

The technique of external cardiac compression

At best this results in a blood flow that is 30% of normal and the exact mechanisms by which these are achieved are unclear. In order to achieve this sort of effect the position of the hands is critical.

1. The rescuer positions himself to one side of the patient.
2. The patient's chest is exposed and the xiphisternum identified. This is the bony prominence in the midline at the junction of the lower borders of the ribs.
3. The index and middle fingers of the rescuer's lower hand are placed on the xiphisternum and, without removing them, the heel of the other hand is placed adjacent to them on the sternum (Figure 5.9a).
4. The fingers are then moved and the heel of the second hand placed on the back of the hand on the sternum. The fingers may then be interlocked (Figure 5.9b).
5. The sternum is then depressed vertically 4–5 cm and then released rapidly. This is repeated at a rate of 80–100/min, with compression and relaxation each taking the same length of time.
6. In order to optimize compression and reduce fatigue, chest compressions should be performed with the rescuer leaning well forward over the patient with straight arms and the hands, elbows and shoulders extended in a straight line. This allows the rescuer to use upper body weight rather than the arm muscles to achieve compression, as they will rapidly tire and reduce efficiency (Figure 5.9b).

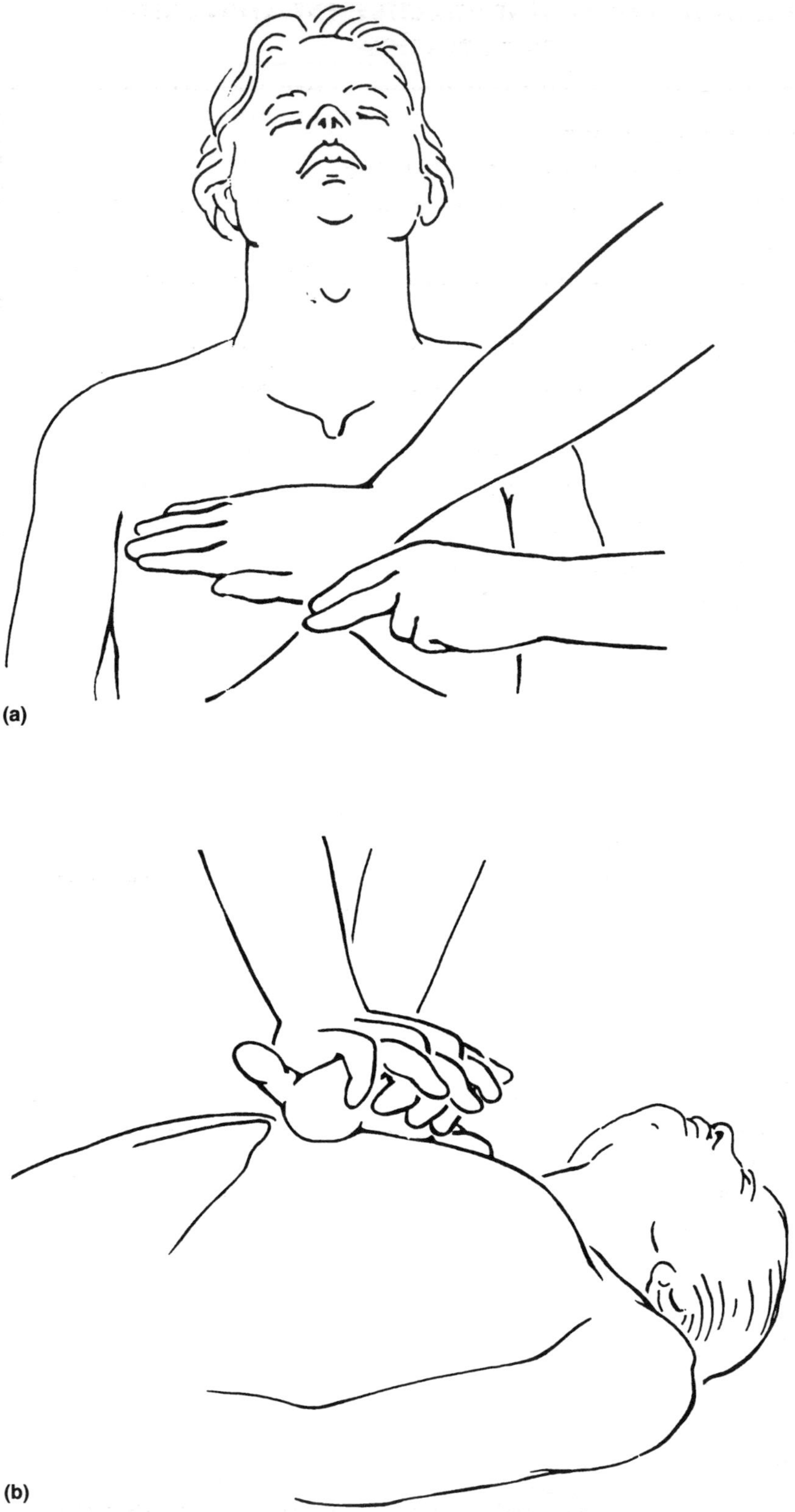

Figure 5.9
(a) Identification of the xiphisternum; (b) external cardiac compression

(a)

(b)

Common causes of ineffective external cardiac compression

1. Wrong hand position:
   Too high: the heart is not compressed
   Too low: the stomach is compressed and risk of aspiration increased
   Too lateral: will injure underlying organs e.g. liver, spleen, bowel.
2. Over-enthusiastic effort: causes cardiac damage, fractures ribs and leads to damage of underlying organs in particular the lungs and the liver.
3. Inadequate effort: usually because the rescuer is not placed high enough above the patient to use his body weight.
4. Failure to release between compressions: prevents venous return and filling of the heart.
5. Inadequate or excessive rate.

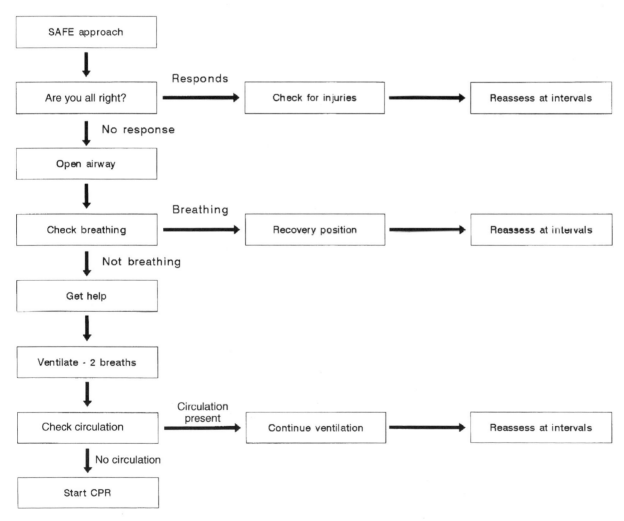

Figure 5.10 The sequence of basic life support

THE RECOVERY POSITION

This is used to help maintain the airway and reduce the risk of aspiration of gastric contents in the unconscious patient who is breathing and has a pulse.

- Place the patient supine, with legs extended, and ensure the airway is open (head tilt, chin lift) (Figure 5.11a).
- Kneeling against the patient, move his closest arm to lie at 90° so that the palm faces upwards.
- Bring the patient's far arm to lie across his chest, so that the back of his hand lies against his cheek (Figure 5.11b).
- Flex the far leg at the hip and knee, keeping the foot on the ground. Grasp the far shoulder (Figure 5.11c).
- Roll the patient, pulling the shoulder towards you, whilst at the same time rotating the upper flexed leg over the lower leg. This is achieved by a combination of pulling on the thigh and gentle downwards pressure.
- Adjust the upper leg so that both hips and knees are flexed to 90° and adjust the hand under the cheek to help maintain the head tilt (Figure 5.11d).
- Finally, check the breathing and pulse regularly.

In this position, gravity helps to maintain a patent airway and allows any vomit or secretions to drain out of the patient's mouth.

If there is **any** suspicion of a spinal injury, then this technique must not be used. Instead, maintain the airway as already described and turn the patient only when there are sufficient people available (usually four) to perform a 'log-roll'.

THE CHOKING PATIENT

Almost any foreign body can cause airway obstruction, although in adults it is usually food, as a result of trying to eat, talk and breathe simultaneously. This has been termed the 'Cafe Coronary'. In these circumstances adults show signs of acute airway obstruction by extreme distress and activity to try and dislodge the obstruction. If obstruction is incomplete, there may be severe coughing and inspiratory stridor.

In a conscious patient who is still able to breathe, encourage coughing. However, if the obstruction is complete or there are signs of exhaustion, then backblows should be used initially.

The rescuer should stand to the side and encourage the patient to lean forwards. The rescuer then supports the patient's chest with

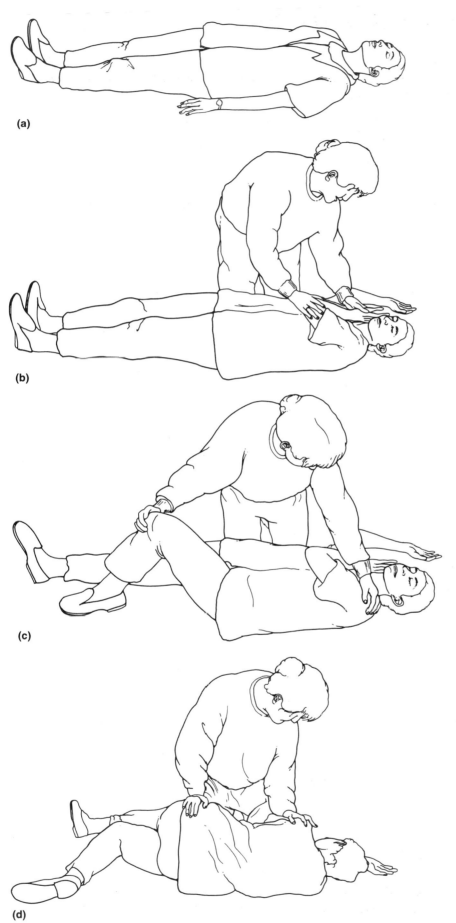

(a)

(b)

(c)

Figure 5.11 The recovery position

(d)

one hand, and then delivers up to five firm blows between the patient's scapulae.

If this fails, then proceed rapidly to the Heimlich manoeuvre.

The Heimlich manoeuvre

This can be performed with the patient standing, sitting or kneeling down. The aim is to expel the foreign body by forcing the diaphragm into the chest and producing a rapid rise in the intrathoracic pressure.

The rescuer should move behind a standing patient and pass both arms around him at the level of the upper abdomen. The rescuer then makes one hand into a fist and places it firmly in the patient's epigastrium. The rescuer's other hand is then placed over the fist and both hands are forced vigorously upwards and backwards (Figure 5.12). This should be repeated 5–10 times, unless the foreign body is dislodged sooner. The Heimlich manoeuvre may force the object into a position where the patient can remove it by coughing or hooking it out with a finger.

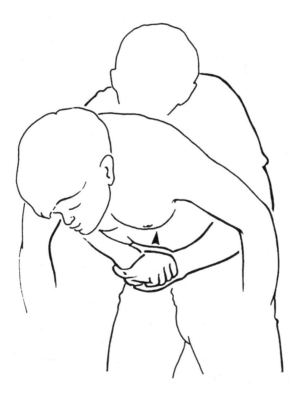

Figure 5.12   The Heimlich manoeuvre

If the patient is unconscious he must be placed supine and a finger sweep attempted. The rescuer should then kneel astride the patient facing his head, and place his hands in the epigastrium as described above. A series of vigorous upward and backward thrusts are used, taking care to apply the pressure in the midline (Figure 5.13).

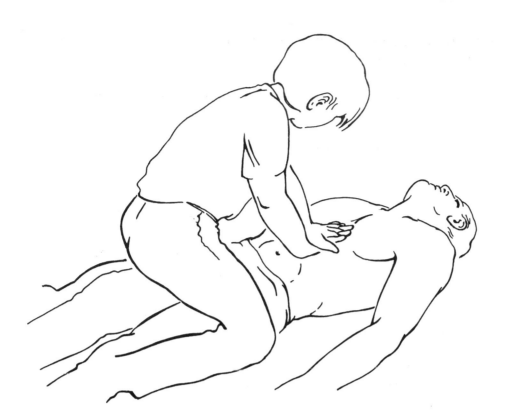

**Figure 5.13
Supine
abdominal
thrusts**

After 5–10 thrusts the airway should be re-inspected and a finger sweep performed to check for any dislodged objects. If this fails to remove the obstruction, two further series of ten thrusts (or alternatively chest thrusts in the style of external cardiac compressions) can be tried.

If all these efforts fail to clear the obstruction, little else can be done without the equipment for either laryngoscopy and intubation or the creation of a surgical airway (cricothyroidotomy) (see Chapters 6 and 14).

SUMMARY

It is essential to acquire the skills of evaluating an unconscious patient, and basic life support before considering the skills of advanced life support. The ability to maintain an airway, perform expired air ventilation and external cardiac compression will significantly improve the outcome for patients who have suffered a cardiac arrest. However, the enthusiasm to help a collapsed patient must not lead to the rescuer placing themselves or anyone else in danger.

6

Airway control and ventilation

In the unconscious patient, prompt assessment and control of the airway along with establishment of ventilation are essential. Failure to perform these simple manoeuvres is a cause of avoidable death. Therefore, in both basic and advanced life support, management of the airway is the first priority – the **A** of 'ABC'.

AIRWAY OBSTRUCTION

Patients have an obstructed airway either as a result of, or cause of their loss of consciousness. The obstruction can occur at many levels:

- Pharynx: by displacement of the tongue, swelling of the epiglottis or soft tissues.

- Larynx: oedema, spasm of the vocal folds (laryngospasm), foreign body, trauma.

- Subglottic: secretions or foreign body, swelling

- Bronchial: bronchospasm, pulmonary oedema, aspiration, pneumothorax.

The most common level of obstruction in the unconscious patient is the pharynx. This has always been thought to be due to a reduction in muscle tone allowing the tongue to fall backwards but this is not the whole explanation as obstruction may still occur when the patient is placed prone. An additional contribution comes from abnormal muscle activity in the pharynx, larynx and neck (Figure 6.1). However, this situation can be rectified and an airway provided by using either head tilt and chin lift or jaw thrust as described in Chapter 5. The success of these actions in providing an airway must then be rapidly assessed using the 'look, listen and feel' approach.

Look at the chest for depth, rate and symmetry of movement. In complete airway obstruction paradoxical movement of the chest and abdomen ('see-sawing') will occur as a result of the increased respiratory effort. In addition, there may be use of accessory muscles. Intercostal and supraclavicular recession may be visible and a tracheal tug may also be apparent. Look also for the presence of abnormal fluids, e.g. blood, gastric contents, frothy sputum (pulmonary oedema). Check the oral cavity for any foreign bodies and finally in the trauma patient look for any wound to the neck or chest.

Listen for breath sounds. Partial obstruction may be accompanied by:

- Inspiratory noises (stridor), which usually indicate upper airway obstruction.

- Expiratory noises, particularly wheezing, which usually suggest obstruction of lower airways as they collapse during expiration.

- 'Crowing', which accompanies laryngeal spasm.

- 'Gurgling', suggesting the presence of liquid or semi-solid material.

- 'Snoring', which usually indicates that the pharynx is still partially occluded by the tongue.

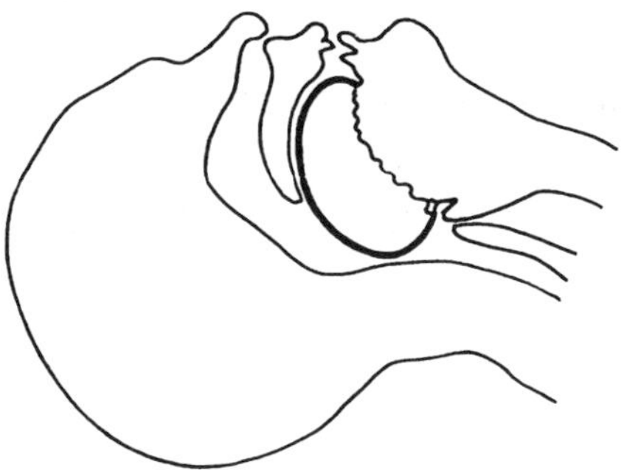

Figure 6.1 Obstruction of the airway by the tongue

Feel for expired air against the side of your cheek, feel for chest movement, comparing one side with the other and finally, if there is any evidence of trauma, feel for the position of the trachea and for any surgical emphysema.

If indicated, a finger sweep can be performed to ensure that obstruction is not due to a foreign body. Broken or very loose dentures should be removed, but well fitting ones may be left in place as they help to maintain the contour of the mouth and make using a bag-mask system easier (see later).

Although the possibility of an injury to the cervical spine must always be borne in mind, the patient is much more likely to die from hypoxia than be rendered quadriplegic as a consequence of carefully conducted airway opening manoeuvres.

AIRWAY ADJUNCTS

These often help to improve or maintain airway patency, either during resuscitation or in a spontaneously breathing patient. Both the oropharyngeal and nasopharyngeal airways are designed to help overcome backward tongue displacement in the unconscious patient. In both cases, however, the head tilt or jaw thrust techniques usually need to be maintained. Details of how to insert airways is discussed in Chapter 14.

Oropharyngeal (Guedel) airways

These are curved plastic tubes, flanged at the oral end and flattened in cross-section so that they can fit between the tongue and the hard palate. They are available in a variety of sizes suitable for all patients, from newborn babies to large adults. The most common sizes are 2–4, for small to large adults respectively. An estimate of the size required can be obtained by comparing the airway with the distance from the corner of the patient's mouth to the angle of the jaw.

Incorrect insertion can push the tongue further back into the pharynx and produce airway obstruction. It can also cause trauma, bleeding and impact unrecognized foreign bodies further into the larynx. Furthermore, in patients who are not deeply unconscious an oral airway may stimulate the pharynx and larynx and cause vomiting and laryngospasm, respectively.

Nasopharyngeal airways

This type of airway is inserted through the patient's nose. They are made from malleable plastic, bevelled at one end, flanged at the other and are round in cross-section to aid insertion. They are sized in millimetres according to their internal diameter and their length increases with diameter. The range of sizes for adults is 6–8 mm, for small to large adults respectively. The thickness of the patient's little finger gives an approximate guide to the nasopharyngeal airway of the correct diameter.

Nasopharyngeal airways are often better tolerated than oropharyngeal airways and may be life-saving in a patient whose mouth cannot be opened – for example one suffering from trismus or maxillary injuries. They should, however, be used with extreme caution if there is suspicion of a fractured base of skull.

Even with careful insertion, bleeding can be precipitated, usually from tissue in the nasopharynx. If the tube is too long, both vomiting and laryngospasm can be induced in patients who are not deeply unconscious.

A further problem associated with both of these types of airway is that during assisted ventilation (see below) air may be directed into the oesophagus. This results in inefficient ventilation of the lungs and causes gastric dilatation. The latter splints the diaphragm, making ventilation difficult, and also predisposes to regurgitation of gastric contents. This is common when high inflation pressures are used. In these circumstances a careful check must always be made to ensure that ventilation is adequate and gastric distension is minimized.

VENTILATORY SUPPORT

If spontaneous ventilation follows airway opening manoeuvres or the insertion of an oro/nasopharyngeal airway, the patient should be placed in an appropriate recovery position (providing there are no contraindications) where there will be less risk of further obstruction (see Chapter 5).

Exhaled air resuscitation

If spontaneous ventilation is inadequate or absent, artificial ventilation must be commenced. If no equipment is available, expired air ventilation will provide 16% oxygen. This can be made more pleasant, and the risks of cross-infection reduced, by the use of simple adjuncts to avoid direct person-to-person contact. An example of this is the Laerdal Pocket Mask. This device has a unidirectional valve to allow expired air to pass to the patient while the patient's expired air is directed away from the rescuer. The mask is transparent to allow the detection of vomit or blood. The more modern version has an additional attachment to allow oxygen supplementation of the rescuer's breath.

Oxygen

Oxygen should be administered to all patients during resuscitation, with the aim of increasing the inspired concentration to 100%. The concentration achieved will depend upon the system used and the flow available. In spontaneously breathing patients, a Venturi mask will deliver a fixed concentration (24–60%) depending upon the mask chosen. A standard concentration mask will deliver up to 60% provided the flow of oxygen is high enough (12–15 l/min). Some patients are more tolerant of nasal cannulae, but these raise the inspired concentration only to approximately 44%. The most effective system is a Hudson mask with a non-rebreathing reservoir, in which the inspired concentration can be raised to 85% with an oxygen flow of 12–15 l/min. This is the most desirable method for use in spontaneously breathing patients.

ADVANCED AIRWAY CONTROL AND VENTILATION

Airway control

The best way of controlling the airway in the deeply unconscious patient is by tracheal intubation. However, the technique requires a greater degree of skill and equipment than the methods already described.

Tracheal intubation may be indicated for a variety of reasons but the most obvious is that all other methods of providing an airway have failed. In addition it allows:

- Suction of and clearance of inhaled debris from the lower respiratory tract.

- Protection against further contamination by regurgitated stomach contents or blood.

- Ventilation to be achieved without leaks, even when airway resistance is high (e.g. in pulmonary oedema, bronchospasm).

- An alternative route for the administration of drugs.

Tracheal intubation

This is the preferred method for controlling the airway during cardiopulmonary resuscitation, for reasons already outlined. Considerable training and practice are required to acquire and maintain the skill of intubation. Repeated attempts by the inexperienced are likely to be unsuccessful, traumatic, compromise oxygenation and delay resuscitation. Intubation can be performed via the oral or nasal route, the former being the most common during CPR.

A list of the equipment required and a description of the technique of orotracheal intubation is given in Chapter 14. Nevertheless, this is not intended as a substitute for practice using a manikin or, better still, an anaesthetized patient under the direction of a skilled anaesthetist.

Tracheal intubation is frequently more difficult to perform during resuscitation. The patient may be awkwardly positioned, equipment may be unfamiliar, assistance limited, CPR obstructive and vomit copious. In these circumstances it is all too easy to persist with the 'almost there' attitude. This must be strongly resisted and if intubation is not successfully accomplished in approximately 30–40 s (about the time one can hold one's breath during the attempt), it should be abandoned and ventilation with 100% oxygen using a bag-valve-mask recommenced before and between any further attempts.

In certain circumstances, e.g. acute epiglottitis, head injury or cervical spine injury, laryngoscopy and attempted intubation are contraindicated because they could lead to deterioration in the patient's condition. In these circumstances, specialist skills, including the use of anaesthetic drugs or fibreoptic laryngoscopy, may be required.

It is not appropriate to learn or practise these techniques during resuscitation.

ALTERNATIVES TO TRACHEAL INTUBATION

Despite the fact that tracheal intubation is at present the optimum method of managing the unconscious patient's airway, for most people acquisition of this skill is time consuming, continuous training unavailable and skill retention poor. Two techniques are now recognized as acceptable alternatives.

The laryngeal mask airway (LMA)

This device consists of a 'mask' which sits over the laryngeal opening, with an inflatable cuff around its perimeter. Attached to the mask is a tube which protrudes from the mouth and through which the patient breathes or is ventilated (Figure 6.2). Although this was originally designed for use in anaesthetized patients breathing spontaneously, patients can be ventilated via the LMA provided that inflation pressures are not excessive. The mask is available in a variety of sizes (1–5) suitable for all patients, from neonates to adults, with sizes 3 to 5 being the most commonly used in female and male adults. The main advantage offered by the LMA is that it can be inserted blindly, and the technique may be more easily mastered than laryngoscopy and tracheal intubation. However, if the mask fails to seal around the larynx or is malpositioned, ventilation is reduced and gastric inflation may occur. Although it does not guarantee against aspiration, the incidence is very low. As with intubation, insertion of an LMA must be preceded whenever possible by a period of pre-oxygenation and any attempt limited to 30–40 s, after which the patient should be ventilated with 100% oxygen using a bag-valve-mask before further attempts.

Despite its limitations, many non-medical personnel are able to insert the LMA more rapidly and successfully than a tracheal tube and achieve more effective ventilation when attached to a bag-valve system than with a facemask. The device has been shown to facilitate ventilation during cardiopulmonary resuscitation and is associated with a very low incidence of aspiration. The LMA is intended for use as an emergency device during CPR, to be replaced when appropriate by a cuffed tracheal tube.

The latest development is the use of the LMA as a conduit to allow the insertion of a tracheal tube to secure the airway in cases of difficult tracheal intubation. The technique of insertion is detailed in Chapter 14.

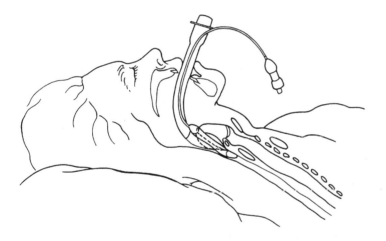

Figure 6.2
Laryngeal mask
in situ

The Combitube

This is the latest in the line of attempts to develop a device which allows ventilation of the lungs and prevents aspiration of any regurgitated gastric contents, yet is capable of blind insertion after minimum training. The Combitube is a double-lumen tube, with a large-volume cuff proximally, a small-volume cuff distally, which combine to provide the functions of an oesophageal obturator and tracheal tube. On insertion the Combitube can pass into either the oesophagus (Figure 14.6a) or trachea (Figure 14.6b). In either situation, ventilation equivalent to using a tracheal tube can be achieved. Currently the Combitube is only manufactured in two sizes – 37 and 41 FG. These can be used in adults taller than 1.5 m

(4'10") and the smaller version in children in whom it would be considered safe to use a cuffed tracheal tube. The main drawback of this device is the cost, coupled with the fact that it is for single use only. Details of the technique of insertion are given in Chapter 14.

Occasionally ventilation and intubation may prove to be impossible using any of the methods described above, usually as a result of obstruction, e.g. glottic oedema, laryngeal trauma or bleeding. In these situations it may be necessary to create a surgical airway below the level of the obstruction. This is usually performed via the cricothyroid membrane using either a large-bore cannula (needle cricothyroidotomy) or a small-diameter tracheostomy tube (surgical cricothyroidotomy). Further details are given in Chapter 14.

An emergency tracheostomy is not appropriate because it is both time consuming and requires considerable surgical skill and equipment.

Although needle cricothyroidotomy allows oxygenation of the patient, carbon dioxide is not eliminated and therefore its usefulness is limited to about 30 min. In addition it is important to note that if the larynx is partially occluded it is essential to allow sufficient time for expiration. Failure to do so will result in increasingly higher intrathoracic pressures which will embarrass venous return, reduce cardiac output and cause pulmonary damage including pneumothoraces.

With a surgical cricothyroidotomy a relatively large-diameter airway is created, and ventilation is more effective than with needle cricothyroidotomy. This allows both oxygenation and elimination of carbon dioxide. In addition, blood and debris can be sucked from the trachea.

Cricoid pressure

This is a manoeuvre used by anaesthetists to prevent regurgitation of gastric contents and pulmonary aspiration during the induction of anaesthesia and intubation of patients with a full stomach.

The cricoid cartilage is a complete ring of cartilage immediately below the thyroid cartilage. Pressure is applied on the cartilage by an assistant, forcing the entire ring backwards, to occlude the oesophagus against the body of the sixth cervical vertebra (Figure 6.3). In so doing it prevents the flow of any gastric contents beyond this point. This manoeuvre is maintained until the tracheal tube is inserted into the larynx, the cuff inflated and the person carrying out the intubation indicates that the pressure can be released.

If a patient starts to vomit the pressure must be released because of the slight risk of rupturing the oesophagus. If pressure is incorrectly applied intubation may be made more difficult.

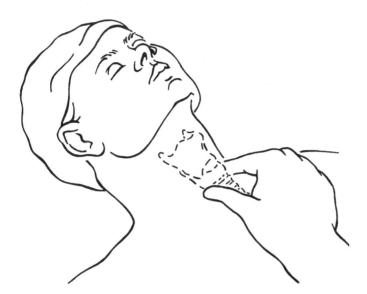

Figure 6.3
Technique for
cricoid pressure

VENTILATION

Whichever device is used to ventilate patients who are apnoeic or breathing inadequately, the ultimate aim is to achieve an inspired oxygen concentration of 100%. The most common device is the self-inflating bag and one-way valve which can be connected to either a facemask or a tracheal tube (Figure 6.4).

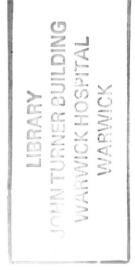

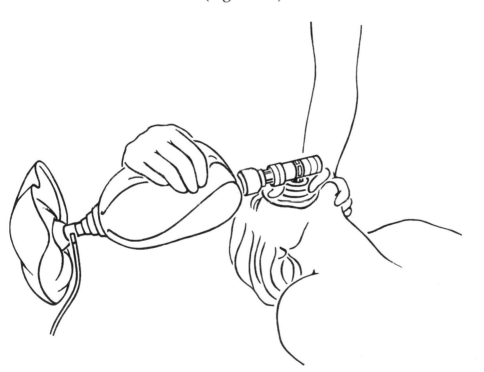

Figure 6.4
Self-inflating
bag-mask and
reservoir

Squeezing the bag delivers its contents to the patient via the one-way valve. On release the bag reinflates, refilling via the inlet valve at the opposite end. At the same time, expired gas from the patient is diverted to the atmosphere via the one-way valve. Using the bag-valve alone (attached to mask or tracheal tube), the patient is ventilated with 21% oxygen, as it refills with ambient air. However, this can (and should) be increased during resuscitation to around 50% by connecting an oxygen supply at 12–15 l/min directly to the bag adjacent to the air intake. If a reservoir bag is also attached, also with an oxygen flow of 12–15 l/min, an inspired oxygen concentration of 95% can be achieved.

Although the self-inflating bag-valve-mask will allow ventilation with higher concentrations of oxygen, it is associated with several problems:

- Considerable skill is required for one person to maintain a gas-tight seal between the mask and the patient's face, whilst at the same time lifting the jaw with one hand and squeezing the bag with the other.

- Any air leak will result in hypoventilation, no matter how energetically the bag is compressed.

- Excessive compression of a bag attached to a facemask results in gas passing into the stomach. This further reduces effective ventilation and increases the risk of regurgitation and aspiration.

- The valve mechanism may become blocked with secretions, vomit or heavy moisture contamination, causing it to stick.

As a result of some of these problems a two-person technique is now recommended during ventilation of a patient with a bag-valve-mask. One person holds the mask in place using both hands as for a pocket mask (Figure 14.3) and an assistant squeezes the bag. In this way a better seal is achieved, the jaw thrust manoeuvre is more easily maintained and the patient can be ventilated more easily.

Clearly these problems can be overcome by tracheal intubation, which eliminates leaks and ensures that oxygen is delivered directly and only into the lungs (always assuming the tube is in the trachea).

Another commonly used method of ventilating patients, via either a facemask or a tracheal tube, is with a Water's circuit (also called a Mapleson C, Westminster Face-piece or rebreathing bag). In this system, the bag is not self-inflating, but refills from a combination of the oxygen supply and air expired from the patient. An adjustable expiratory valve is also provided, situated between the bag and the mask/tube connection. By almost closing this valve, it appears possible to ventilate patients adequately with a low flow of oxygen (4 l/min) as judged by chest movement and listening to breath sounds. However, the bag is filling predominantly with expired air and as a result carbon dioxide accumulates. The patient is then ventilated, or rebreathes, expired gas containing ever higher concentrations of carbon dioxide and rapidly becomes hypercarbic. This is clearly undesirable during resuscitation, especially if the patient has raised intracranial pressure from any cause.

A high flow of oxygen must always be used with this system (12–15 l/min) to flush out expired air and ensure that the bag fills with oxygen.

The ultimate method of ventilating patients during resuscitation is to use a mechanical ventilator. When using these devices the most important feature to remember is that they are good servants, but poor masters. They will do only what they are set to do, and will not automatically compensate for changes in the patient's condition during resuscitation. It is imperative therefore that they are set correctly and checked regularly when used.

A variety of small portable ventilators are used during resuscitation (e.g. pneuPAC) and are generally gas powered. If an oxygen cylinder is used as both the supply of respiratory gas and the power for the ventilator, its contents will be used more rapidly. This is of particular importance if a patient is being transported over long distances because adequate oxygen supplies must be taken.

Gas-powered portable ventilators are classified as time cycled and often have a fixed inspiratory:expiratory ratio. They provide a constant flow of gas during inspiration and expiration occurs passively to the atmosphere. The volume delivered depends on the inspiratory time (i.e. longer times, larger breaths) with the pressure in the airway rising during inspiration. As a safety feature, these devices can often be 'pressure limited' by a relief valve opening to protect the lungs against excessive pressures (barotrauma).

A ventilator should initially be set to deliver 10 ml/kg at a rate of 12 breaths/min. Some ventilators have co-ordinated markings on the controls to facilitate rapid initial setting for patients of different sizes. The correct setting will ultimately be determined by analysis of arterial blood gases.

Care should be taken when using ventilators with relief valves fixed to open at relatively low pressures. The pressure may be exceeded during CPR as a chest compression coincides with a breath from the ventilator, resulting in inadequate ventilation. By the same mechanism ventilators with adjustable pressure relief valves, if set too high, may subject patients to excessively high pressures. These risks can be reduced by decreasing the rate of ventilation (breaths/min) to allow co-ordination of breaths and compressions.

If there is any doubt about the performance of the ventilator, the safest option is to temporarily disconnect it and use a self-inflating bag-valve assembly with oxygen and reservoir until skilled help is available.

SUCTION

Once the trachea has been intubated (orally or by a surgical airway) suction should be performed to remove secretions, vomit or blood. This must be carried out carefully to avoid making the patient hypoxic and bradycardic and can be performed in the following way:

- The patient is ventilated with 100% oxygen.

- Wearing gloves, the operator introduces a sterile catheter through the airway into the trachea without suction.

- The diameter of the catheter should be less than half that of the tracheal tube or surgical airway.

- Suction is commenced and the catheter withdrawn using a rotating motion over 10–15 s.

- Irrespective of the amount of blood/mucus removed, the catheter must not be reintroduced without a further period of oxygenation.

- Tenacious secretions can be loosened by prior instillation of 10 ml sterile saline followed by five vigorous manual ventilations. Suction is then performed as above.

Suction must not be applied directly to the tracheal tube or surgical airway, as this will result in life-threatening hypoxia and dysrhythmias.

SUMMARY

Airway control and ventilation are essential prerequisites for successful cardiopulmonary resuscitation. Recognition of airway obstruction, its correction and the commencement of artificial ventilation should be carried out initially using basic techniques of which AnyBody is Capable. It should not be delayed by the unavailability of equipment. Tracheal intubation remains the best method of securing and controlling the airway, but requires additional equipment, skill and practice. The ultimate aim is to ventilate the patient with 100% oxygen. Occasionally, when all other methods of ventilation have failed, a surgical airway may be required as a life-saving procedure.

———7———
Access to the circulation

Objectives

After reading this chapter you should be able to:

- Identify the anatomy for peripheral and central venous cannulation
- Be familiar with the technique used for peripheral, central venous and intraosseous cannulation
- Recognize the complications associated with these techniques

VENOUS ACCESS

Venous access is an essential part of advanced life support. Once successful it allows drugs and fluids to be given to complete the 'chain of survival'. Venous cannulation is an invasive procedure which must not be treated with complacency.

Intravenous (IV) access can be achieved via several routes:

1. Percutaneous cannulation of a peripheral vein.
2. Following surgical exposure of a vein in the 'cutdown' technique.
3. Percutaneous cannulation of a central vein.
4. Intraosseous route.

Success is optimized and complications minimized when the operator has:

- Knowledge of the local anatomy.
- Familiarity with equipment.
- Understanding of the technique.
- Awareness of complications.

PERIPHERAL VENOUS CANNULATION

This is most commonly performed in the antecubital fossa.

The cephalic vein passes through the antecubital fossa on the lateral side and the basilic vein enters the antecubital fossa very medially – just in front of the medial epicondyle of the elbow. These two large veins are joined by the **median cubital** or **antecubital vein**. The median vein of the forearm also drains into the basilic vein (Figure 7.1).

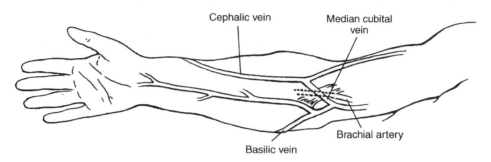

**Figure 7.1
Veins of the forearm and antecubital fossa**

Although the veins in this area are prominent and easily cannulated, there are many other adjacent vital structures which can be easily damaged.

By far the most popular device for achieving peripheral intravenous access is the cannula over needle, available in a wide variety of sizes from 12 to 27 gauge (g). It consists of a plastic (PTFE or similar material) cannula which is mounted on a smaller-diameter metal needle, the bevel of which protrudes from the cannula. The other end of the needle is attached to a transparent 'flashback chamber', which fills with blood when the needle bevel lies within the vein. Some devices have flanges or 'wings' to facilitate attachment to the skin. All cannulae have a standard luer-lock fitting for attaching a giving set and some have a valved injection port through which drugs can be administered.

Details of the technique of insertion are given in Chapter 15.

Complications

- Failed cannulation is the most common, usually as a result of pushing the needle completely through the vein. Incidence is inversely related to experience.

- Haematomas are usually secondary to the above if inadequate pressure is applied to prevent blood leaking from the vein. They are made worse by forgetting to remove the tourniquet!

- Extravasation of fluid or drugs is commonly a result of failing to recognize that the cannula is not within the vein before use. Placing a cannula over a joint or prolonged use to infuse fluids under pressure also predispose to leakage. Once this problem has been identified, the cannula must no longer be used.

Damage to the overlying tissues will depend primarily upon the nature of the extravasated fluid.

- Damage to other local structures is secondary to poor technique and lack of knowledge of the local anatomy.

- Air embolus occurs when the pressure in the veins is lower than in the right side of the heart and air is entrained. It is usually prevented from occurring by the peripheral veins collapsing as they empty. However, once a cannula is in place collapse is prevented.

- The plastic cannula can be sheared, and fragments may enter the circulation. This is usually a result of trying to reintroduce the needle after it has been withdrawn. The safest action is to withdraw the whole cannula and attempt cannulation at another site.

- The needle may fracture as a result of careless manipulation with the finer cannulae. Surgical intervention is needed to remove the fragment.

- Inflammation of the vein (thrombophlebitis) is related to the length of time the vein is in use and amount of irritation caused by the substances flowing through it. High concentrations of drugs, fluids with extremes of pH or high osmolality are the main causes. Once a vein shows signs of thrombophlebitis (it becomes tender, red and flow deteriorates), the cannula must be removed to prevent infection or thrombosis which may spread proximally.

CUTDOWN

Occasionally is it not possible to cannulate a peripheral vein percutaneously. This is not uncommon in patients who have arrested in electromechanical dissociation. If the skills are not available to obtain central venous access an alternative is to cannulate a vein under direct vision. The vein most commonly used is the long saphenous at the ankle.

This vein is very consistent in its location, 2 cm in front of and 2 cm above the medial malleolus (Figure 7.2). However, it is accompanied very closely by the saphenous nerve. An alternative is the median cubital vein in the antecubital fossa.

The vein is exposed and a small hole made in to accept a cannula which is advanced up the vein, secured in place and the wound closed and dressed appropriately.

Details of this technique are given in Chapter 15.

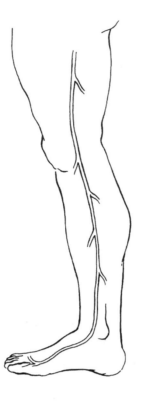

**Figure 7.2
Course of the
saphenous vein**

Complications

- Inability to identify the vein.

- Transection of the vein or adjacent structures.

- Haematoma formation.

- Venous thrombosis.

- Infection.

CENTRAL VENOUS CANNULATION

Cannulation of peripheral veins is not the ideal form of venous access following a cardiac arrest because the procedure can be time consuming and the drug transit time from the periphery to the heart is prolonged. Therefore, catheterization of a central vein is recommended and, paradoxically, relatively easy to perform. However, in the circumstances of a cardiac arrest, it may be necessary for someone without a great deal of experience to catheterize a central vein safely and quickly. Therefore a technique is required which is easy to perform, as well as having a high success rate with few complications. Details of the technique used are given in Chapter 15.

The two most common routes used to gain access to the central veins are the internal jugular vein and subclavian vein. The relationship of these veins is shown in Figure 7.3.

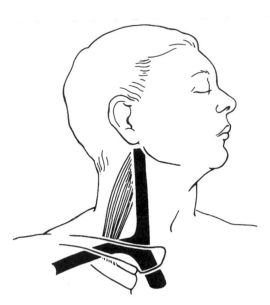

Figure 7.3 The course of the central veins of the neck

The main advantage of the subclavian vein is that it is prevented from collapsing by the surrounding tissues and therefore is more easily identified in shocked and cardiac arrest patients. However, there are many potential complications of this route and the internal jugular vein is becoming increasingly more popular because of its relative safety.

Two main techniques are used for cannulation of the central veins. A cannula over needle can be used in a similar manner to that described for peripheral veins. The main difference is that the cannula is usually longer – approximately 15 cm. Increasingly more popular is the Seldinger technique.

Seldinger technique

The vein chosen is entered percutaneously with a small-gauge pilot needle attached to a syringe. When blood can be freely aspirated, the syringe is removed and a flexible wire is inserted through the needle for a distance of 5–6 cm into the vein. The needle is then carefully removed, leaving the wire behind. The cannula is loaded onto the wire, ensuring that the distal end of the wire protrudes from the cannula. The cannula and wire are then advanced into the vein, the distal end of the wire being held to ensure that it does not slip into the vein. The wire is removed and a syringe attached to the cannula; blood is aspirated to confirm that the cannula is in the vein.

If during the procedure the wire does not pass easily into the vein, the needle and wire should be withdrawn together and the procedure started afresh.

A modification of the Seldinger technique is the passage of a Teflon dilator along the guidewire ahead of the cannula. This dilator facilitates the passage of a very large bore (e.g. 8 FG) intravenous cannula which can be used for rapid infusion or the insertion of transvenous pacing wires.

Complications of subclavian vein cannulation

- **Pneumothorax**: the dome of the pleura lies above the level of the clavicle and is easily punctured if the needle is advanced at too deep an angle. Bilateral attempts are not recommended.
- **Haemothorax**: usually from puncture of the subclavian artery or more rarely tearing of the vein.
- **Brachial plexus injury**: needle inserted in the wrong direction.
- **Tracheal puncture**: needle inserted too far.
- **Infection**: usually at site of entry, due to poor aseptic technique.

Complications of internal jugular cannulation

- **Failure**: usually because the initial attempt is made too far laterally.
- **Haematoma**: due to puncture of the carotid artery. Fortunately this is less of a problem with the Seldinger technique as pressure can be applied to the artery to minimize bleeding.
- **Pneumothorax**: rare, as the vein is well above the pleura (unless too long a needle is used!).
- **Puncture of vertebral vessels, oesophagus, trachea**: rare, as these structures are medial to the carotid artery.

Because of the danger with either technique of creating a pneumothorax, which, if unrecognized, may tension, a chest radiograph must always be obtained at the earliest opportunity. This rule applies even if the attempt has been unsuccessful.

INTRAOSSEOUS ROUTE

Percutaneous venous cannulation is often technically more difficult in children, particularly when they are critically ill. The intraosseous route provides rapid and effective access to the circulation in children. It allows the administration of fluids and drugs, with levels of the latter being comparable to those achieved when given via a central vein. Furthermore, aspirated marrow can be used to cross-match blood in the absence of a blood sample. It is a technique most suited to children less than six years of age, as beyond this age the vascular red marrow is gradually replaced by fatty yellow marrow.

The proximal tibia is the most commonly used site for intraosseous access: on the anterior surface 2–3 cm below the tibial tuberosity. Alternatively the anterior surface of the femur, 3 cm above the lateral condyle, can be used (Figure 7.4).

These sites are relatively free of other local important structures. The most relevant feature to be borne in mind is the proximity of the growth plates (epiphyses). If these are damaged, subsequent bone growth and development could be affected.

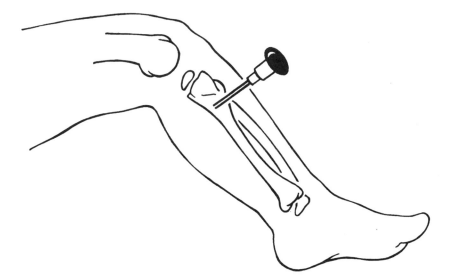

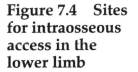

Figure 7.4 Sites for intraosseous access in the lower limb

Details of the technique are given in Chapter 15.

If neither lower limb can be used, the upper limb is used. The site of puncture is the distal humerus, just proximal to the lateral epicondyle.

Although bone marrow biopsy needles can be used, needles are now specifically produced for this procedure. As they have to pierce the bone cortex they are made entirely of metal. They come in a variety of designs, but they all have certain features in common. The needles have a short shaft, with a central solid trocar, which has a relatively large handle attached. The trocar must be unscrewed before it can be removed from the needle. The external end of the needle has a standard luer-lock fitting. Some needles have a screw thread to improve their security in the bone. These needles come in a range of sizes: 16–20 g for children less than 18 months, 12–16 g for children older than 18 months.

Complications

Fortunately these are very rare and mainly theoretical.

- Failure to enter the bone marrow cavity is the most common problem. This may occur more often when the distal femur is used due to the difficulty in identifying the correct landmarks.

- If the needle is incorrectly placed, fluid may extravasate and if prolonged this could cause a compartment syndrome.

- Infection in the skin, abscess formation and ultimately osteomyelitis may occur, but appear to be related to prolonged use of a needle.

- Fat and marrow emboli can occur, particularly if excessive pressure is used to infuse drugs or fluid.

- Damage to the growth plate of the bone used could result from careless placement and in very young children a fracture could occur if excessive force is used.

Intraosseous access to the circulation is a life-saving procedure and not a definitive route for resuscitation of a sick child. Once alternative routes of venous access have been achieved, the intraosseous needle should be removed.

SUMMARY

Access to the circulation allows the completion of the final link in the 'chain of survival'. If peripheral venous access is already available, and functioning adequately, it can be used initially but early consideration must be given to establishing central venous access. In children, early consideration should be given to using the intraosseous route rather than persisting unsuccessfully with other routes.

8

Cardiac monitoring and rhythm recognition

Objectives

After reading this chapter you should be able to:

- Understand the origin and passage of the electrical activity in the heart

- Recognize patients for whom this activity should be monitored and how it should be carried out

- Understand the system for analysing electrical activity recorded on a rhythm strip

CARDIAC ELECTRICAL ACTIVITY: ITS ORIGIN AND ORGANIZATION

The sino-atrial node (SAN) is a specialized area of cardiac muscle which generates a continuous sequence of regularly timed waves of electrical activity known as depolarization. These radiate through both atria, inducing contraction. As the depolarization spreads through the atria it also gives rise to the P wave on the electrocardiogram (ECG). Normally the P wave has a duration of 0.08–0.12 s.

Atrial depolarization normally finishes by converging on a specialized collection of cells called the atrioventricular node (AVN) located at the base of the right atrium. This delays the transmission of the depolarizing wave to the ventricles and gives rise to a significant proportion of the PR interval. The latter is measured on the ECG tracing from the start of the P wave to the first deflection of the QRS complex.

From the AVN, the wave of depolarization is conducted through the fibrous atrioventricular barrier via the bundle of His. At the proximal part of the muscular intraventricular septum this splits into the right and left bundle branches, with the latter subsequently separating into anterior and posterior divisions (fascicles). These, in turn, terminate into small (Purkinje) fibres which transmit the electrical impulse to the non-specialized ventricular myocardium. The passage of the impulse through the specialized ventricular conduction system is rapid compared to the AVN and is represented by the QRS wave on the ECG.

Following stimulation, the myocardial cells recover their normal resting electrical potential in an active biochemical process called repolarization. The atrial repolarization wave is usually obscured by the QRS, but the ventricular repolarization gives rise to the T wave. For most of the period of repolarization the ventricles remain unresponsive (or 'refractory') to further electrical stimulation. A diagrammatic representation of the conducting system and its relationship to the ECG is shown in Figure 8.1.

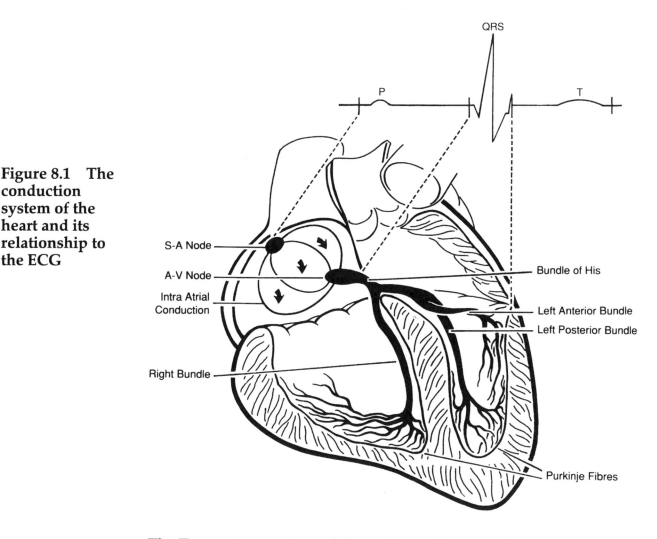

Figure 8.1 The conduction system of the heart and its relationship to the ECG

The T wave is sometimes followed by a U wave, which is a rounded deflection in the same direction as the T wave. Its exact genesis is unclear but it becomes more prominent in hypokalaemia and hypercalcaemia and inverted in ischaemic heart disease.

The QT interval is measured from the beginning of the QRS complex to the end of the T wave. Consequently it represents the total time for ventricular depolarization and repolarization. Prolongation of this interval is mainly associated with clinical conditions which delay ventricular repolarization. The significance of a prolonged QT interval is that it increases the period of time where the ventricles are susceptible to lethal dysrhythmias (see later).

It is important to realize that the duration of the QT interval is inversely dependent on the heart rate, and directly dependent on age and gender. The corrected QT interval (QTc) is obtained once heart rate has been taken into account (normal range 0.35–0.42 s). Fortunately many diagnostic ECG machines carry out this calculation automatically.

PATHOLOGY OF THE CONDUCTING SYSTEM

The origin and spread of depolarization through the heart can be affected by ischaemic disease, drugs, trauma and abnormal metabolic conditions. This can lead to the depolarization originating from abnormal areas of the heart and spreading by an atypical route. The ECG can be used in these situations to help to locate the affected sites.

All parts of the special conducting system have the ability to initiate a wave of depolarization but do so at varying frequencies. The eventual heart rate is determined by that part of the conducting system which has the fastest intrinsic rate of depolarization, normally the SAN. After the SAN, the next fastest part is usually the atria. If this is also defective the AVN will take over as the cardiac pacemaker, followed in turn by the bundle of His and the ventricular myocardium.

Occasionally a pathological focus which has a faster intrinsic rate of depolarization than the SAN develops in the heart. As a consequence, this focus will replace the SAN as the cardiac pacemaker.

CAUSES OF DYSRHYTHMIA

Increasing the heart rate

An increase in heart rate occurs normally as a result of emotion, exercise and fear. These are mediated by the sympathetic nervous system acting on the SAN to increase its rate of depolarization. However, an increase in the heart rate can also result from the following pathological reasons:

- Automaticity
- Re-entry
- Both

Automaticity

Automaticity is the ability to depolarize spontaneously, and is a common feature of cells in the conducting system and certain areas of myocardium. As mentioned previously, the SAN usually has the fastest rate of depolarization and therefore acts as the dominant pacemaker.

Re-entry

Re-entry occurs when there is a dual conducting system between the atria and the ventricles. This can be either within the AVN or bypassing it (e.g. Wolff–Parkinson–White and Lown–Ganong–Levine syndromes). One pathway (A) has a unidirectional block (or a longer refractory period) and the other (B) has a slow conduction rate (Figure 8.2).

Figure 8.2 The origin of a circus movement

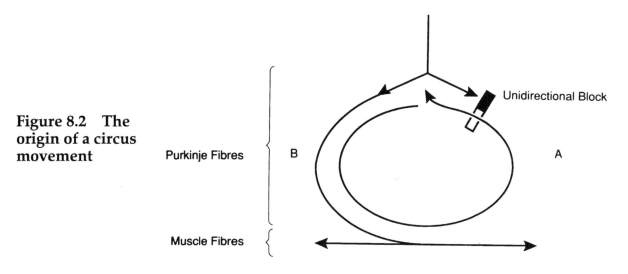

In response to a premature beat, the impulse has to go down the slow pathway (B). This is because the fast pathway (A) has not repolarized from the previous beat and is therefore unable to conduct the electrical impulse. This increase in transit time allows A to repolarize so that the impulse can be conducted opposite to the normal direction of flow. This gives B sufficient time to repolarize and so be able to be stimulated by the retrograde impulse which has travelled along A. Consequently a self-sustaining cycle of electrical impulses is created.

Both

Automaticity and re-entry can act together.

Slowing of the heart rate

A reduction in the heart rate is a normal physiological response during sleep and at rest in the athletic individual. The heart rate can also fall in certain pathological conditions in which the intrinsic rate of depolarization of the intrinsic cardiac pacemaker and/or the conducting system are reduced. Ischaemic heart disease is the most common cause but drugs, trauma and other diseases can also be responsible.

MONITORING CARDIAC ELECTRICAL ACTIVITY

In the acute situation cardiac electrical activity is usually continuously assessed by an ECG monitor connected to the patient by a standard system of electrical leads.

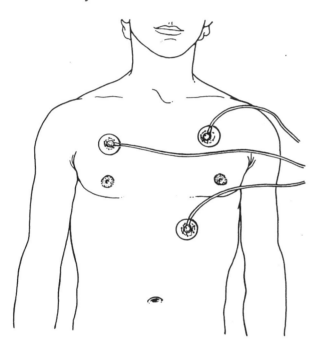

**Figure 8.3
Monitoring the
electrocardiogram**

Cardiac ECG monitors

Though there are many different types of cardiac monitor, most have certain features in common: there is a screen for displaying the cardiac rhythm and a device for obtaining a copy of it. This printout is commonly known as the 'rhythm strip'. Most models also incorporate a heart rate meter which is triggered by the QRS complexes and a device to automatically store a record of the ECG if the heart rate falls outside certain preset limits. Lights and audible signals may provide additional indications of the heart rate.

Traditional (analogue) monitors display the ECG trace on a cathode ray oscilloscope screen, whereas more modern machines tend to convert the electronic signal into digital form. The more modern machines perform complex functions such as computer-aided rhythm analysis, automatic and semi-automatic defibrillation (see Chapter 16) and electronic storage of the signal for later playback and analysis.

Leads

Lead I measures the voltage between the right and left shoulder. It gives a good view of the left lateral aspect of the heart and the QRS complex but does not necessarily give a good picture of the P wave (Figure 8.4).

Lead II measures the voltage between the right shoulder and left leg. It is the lead most commonly used for monitoring the cardiac rhythm. As it is in line with the mean frontal cardiac axis, it gives a good view of both the QRS and P wave. It also shows shifts in the direction of the axis (Figure 8.4).

Lead III measures the voltage between the left shoulder and left lower chest (or leg). It is rarely an advantage in dysrhythmia recognition but it does give a good view of the inferior aspect of the heart (Figure 8.4).

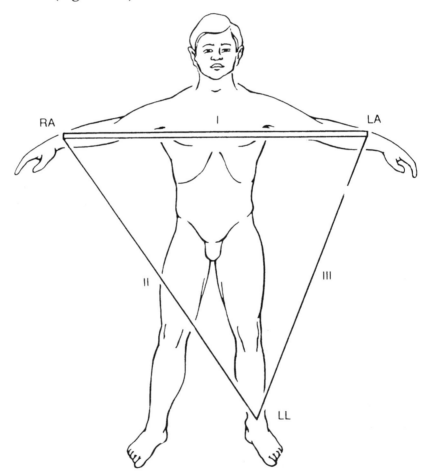

Figure 8.4   The bipolar limb leads

The remaining leads are not used during routine monitoring or the initial management of a cardiac arrest; they are, however, required for definitive dysrhythmia analysis and determining the position of the cardiac axis. The MCL1 lead measures the voltage between the right pectoral area (V1 position) and the left shoulder. This gives a good view of the QRS and P wave, but it is not commonly used.

Leads I, II, III, and aVR, aVL, aVF look at the heart in the vertical plane (Figure 8.5).

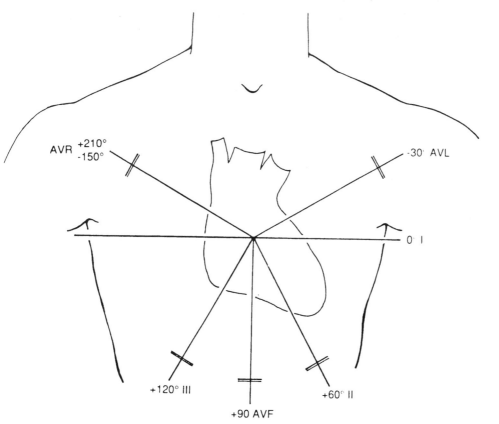
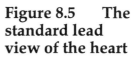

Figure 8.5 The standard lead view of the heart

Leads V1–6 view the heart in the horizontal plane: V1 and V2 look at the right ventricle, V3 and V4 the interventricular septum and V5 and V6 mainly the left ventricle (Figure 8.6).

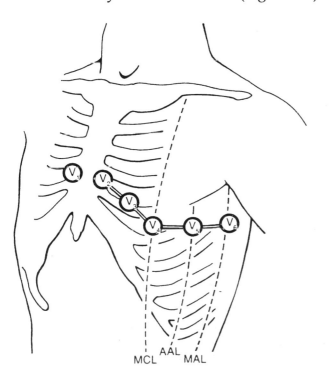

Figure 8.6 The chest leads

Practical points

- The ECG monitor should be used on all patients presenting with chest pain, syncope, dizziness, collapse, hypotension, palpitations and cardiac arrest.

- ECG machines record at a standard speed of 25 mm/s. Calibrated recording paper is used so that each large square (5 mm) is equivalent to 0.2 s and each small square to 0.04 seconds. The amplitude of the trace is standardized at 1 millivolt per centimetre (1 mV/cm) and most machines have the capability of testing this (Figure 8.7).

Figure 8.7 Voltage calibration of the electrocardiogram

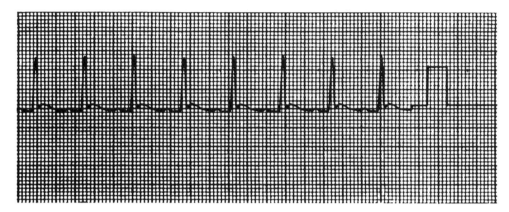

- To minimize electrical interference the electrodes should be all of the same type, applied over bone rather than muscle and positioned equidistant from one another. Hair should be removed from the areas where the electrodes are to be attached and the skin cleaned with alcohol to dissolve surface oil. The electrodes should be positioned on the patient's chest so that they will not interfere with any other activities such as external cardiac massage.

- Adhesive silver/silver chloride electrodes give the best signal and, if readily available, are preferable to defibrillation paddles even for the first 'quick look' in cardiac arrest. Another advantage is that paddles will give a reading only when they are in position and therefore are not practical for continuously assessing the rhythm. If paddles are used, it is essential that they are placed over gel pads so that electrical contact can be facilitated.

- Ensure that the QRS height is sufficient to stimulate the rate meter by adjusting the gain control. However, this should not be so excessive as to cause artefacts on the monitor.

- Any activity, such as drug administration or carotid sinus massage, should be recorded on the rhythm strip as it happens. This helps greatly in the later analysis of the dysrhythmia.

- A common artefact seen is that produced by the patient moving, undergoing strenuous respiratory effort or being subjected to external cardiac compression. As the last is usually sufficient to completely mask the patient's own cardiac rhythm, it must be stopped for 1–2 s so that the cardiac arrest rhythm can be analysed (see later).

- It is important to realize that the leads used to monitor dysrhythmias are **not** the optimum ones for recording changes in the ST segment and T wave. A 'diagnostic' setting may be required to accurately reproduce ST displacement but this produces more baseline wandering.

- If time permits, old notes should be obtained, previous ECGs studied and a full 12-lead ECG should be carried out as this helps with dysrhythmia analysis.

A SYSTEMATIC APPROACH TO INTERPRETING A RHYTHM STRIP

Avoid the temptation to simply 'eyeball' the rhythm strip produced by the ECG monitor. Develop a system so that clues and multiple problems are not missed.

Basic principles

It is helpful to remember the following basic principle when you are interpreting the rhythm strip:

- If the depolarization wave is moving towards the electrode then an upward (positive) deflection is seen on the monitor.

- If the depolarization wave is moving away from the electrode then a downward (negative) deflection is seen on the monitor.

Box 8.1 contains one of the many systems which has been developed for health care workers interpreting a rhythm strip from lead II in the acute situation. It is an effective system based upon a series of questions which pick out the most life-threatening dysrhythmias first.

How is the patient?

Always remember – treat the patient, not the rhythm

It is extremely important to see the patient before making a diagnosis and suggesting a treatment from a single rhythm strip. For example, a patient who is not breathing and has no palpable pulse is suffering from a cardiorespiratory arrest irrespective of what the monitor shows. For example, if the arrest occurs despite normal (or

Box 8.1   Systematic approach to interpreting a rhythm strip

How is the patient?

Is there any electrical activity?

      No: Asystole
      Yes: Not asystole

Are there recognizable complexes?

      No: Ventricular fibrillation
      Yes: Not ventricular fibrillation

What is the ventricular rate?

What is the rhythm?

      Regular
      Regular irregularity
      Irregular irregularity

Are the P waves uniform?

      Shape
      Timing: early or later than normal?

Is there atrial flutter?

Are there the same number of P waves as QRS complexes?

      Yes: What is the PR interval?
      No: Is the PR interval constant?
             Is the RR interval constant?

Is the QRS duration normal?

      Yes: Normal ventricular conduction
      No: Abnormal ventricular conduction:
                Shape
                Timing: early or later than normal?
                Frequency

          Ventricular tachycardia:
                SVT with aberrant ventricular conduction
                Torsade de pointes

          Idioventricular rhythm:
                Agonal rhythm

near normal) electrical activity then **electromechanical dissociation** exists.

Is there any electrical activity?

If there is no electrical activity check:

Connections: to monitor, to patient

QRS gain

Leads I and III

If there is still no electrical activity diagnose **asystole** (Figure 8.8). However, beware that a completely flat tracing, without any baseline wandering, is usually caused by the patient's leads not being connected to the monitor.

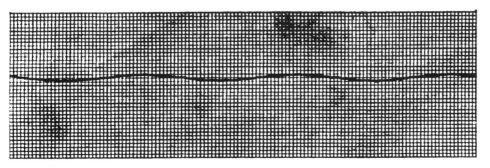

**Figure 8.8
Asystole**

Occasionally P waves can be detected, indicating that atrial activity is still present. This usually occurs, transiently, shortly after the onset of ventricular asystole and is associated with a better prognosis than when P waves are absent.

Are there any recognizable complexes?

If there are no recognizable complexes diagnose **ventricular fibrillation** (VF) (Figure 8.9).

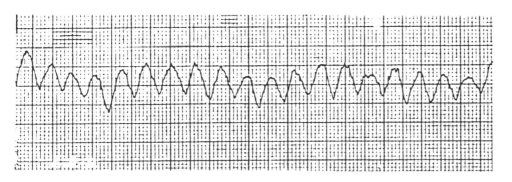

**Figure 8.9
Ventricular
fibrillation**

VF gives rise to a totally chaotic rhythm because small areas of the myocardium depolarize in a random fashion. Initially the amplitude of the waveform is large and the dysrhythmia is known as 'coarse

VF'. Over time 'fine VF' develops because the amplitude diminishes and the tracing becomes flatter. Eventually asystole results.

It is often difficult to determine when the patient has made the transition from fine VF to asystole. This is made more difficult by the presence of any baseline wandering, electrical interference and movement of the patient. In such cases the rhythm should be repeated, taking the precautions listed for asystole. In addition all contact with the patient should cease briefly (less than 5 s) so that a reliable tracing can be gained without interference.

The presence or absence of the most common cardiac arrest rhythms will have been determined by answering these first three questions. As these require immediate treatment (see Chapter 9), further interpretation of the ECG assumes that these rhythms have been excluded.

What is the ventricular rate?

Rate = 300/number of large squares between consecutive R waves. Figure 8.10 demonstrates a ventricular rate of 75 beats/min.

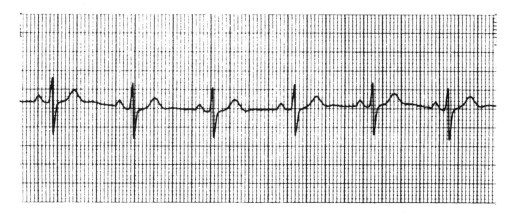

Figure 8.10 Sinus rhythm: rate 75 beats/min

Any rhythm which has a ventricular rate greater than 100 is called a **tachycardia**. A common type is a **sinus tachycardia** which has, by definition, one P wave before each QRS and usually has a rate of 100–130 beats/min (Figure 8.11). In contrast, a ventricular rate less than 60/min is called a **bradycardia**. **Sinus bradycardia** is a common type of bradycardia which has, like its fast namesake, a P wave before each QRS.

Supraventricular tachycardias (SVT) (Figure 8.12) can be divided into two groups depending upon whether they result from re-entry or enhanced automaticity. However, in the absence of an atrial premature beat (see later) prior to the tachycardia commencing, it is

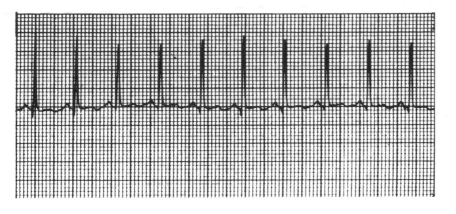

**Figure 8.11
Sinus
tachycardia: rate
136 beats/min**

not possible on routine ECG monitoring to distinguish between these groups.

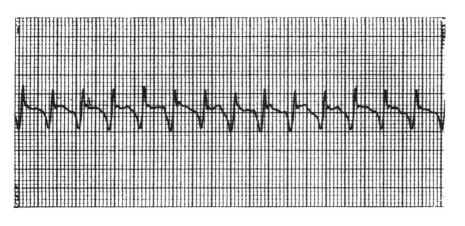

**Figure 8.12
Supraventricular
tachycardia**

The QRS complexes are narrow with this condition unless there is an aberrant conduction through the ventricles producing widening of the QRS complex (see later).

What is the rhythm?

To answer this question correctly it is important to carefully inspect an adequate length of the rhythm strip tracing. In this way it will be possible to detect subtle variations in rhythm.

Assessment of the regularity of the rhythm of the R waves is made by comparing the RR intervals of adjacent beats at different places in the tracing. Callipers or dividers are very useful for this but it is also possible to obtain an accurate result by marking the peaks of four adjacent R waves on a piece of paper. This must be done precisely because rhythm irregularity becomes less marked as the heart rate increases. The paper is then moved along the strip to see if the gaps correspond. If they do then the rhythm is regular. As interpretation of a fast heart rate can be difficult, a further rhythm strip recorded during carotid sinus massage may help by temporarily slowing the heart rate.

A **sinus rhythm** is diagnosed when:

- The P waves have a normal duration.
- The PR interval has a normal and consistent duration (0.12–0.2 s).
- The heart rate is between 60 and 100/min.
- A P wave precedes each QRS complex.

Usually successive RR intervals are constant but occasionally, in healthy young individuals, the RR interval varies with respiration. Nevertheless the P wave shape and PR interval remains the same. This variation in the RR interval is called **sinus arrhythmia** and results from impairment of the cardio-inhibitory centre during inspiration causing the heart rate to increase. The opposite occurs during expiration.

If the RR interval is irregular, it is important to decide whether it is an 'irregular irregularity', i.e. with no recognizable pattern, or a 'regular irregularity', i.e. the variation repeats in a regular fashion. In the latter case the relationship between the P waves and the QRS waves assumes special importance (this will be discussed in greater detail later).

When an irregular irregularity in the RR interval is associated with a constant QRS shape, a likely diagnosis is **atrial fibrillation** (AF) (Figure 8.13).

Figure 8.13
Atrial fibrillation

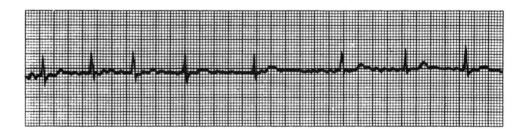

AF is due to atrial depolarization in a disorganized fashion at a rate of 350–600/min with conduction through the AVN occurring at an irregular rate. There are no P waves with AF, but the baseline may vary between fine and coarse fluctuations in different parts of the strip.

Are the P waves uniform?

Normal P waves have a duration of 0.08–0.12 s (two to three little squares) and a vertical deflection less than 2.5 mm. They can be distinguished from the larger T waves, which have a duration of 0.28 s (seven little squares).

It is important to check the whole strip for P waves because they may be hidden in the QRS complex or T wave, producing inconsistent and abnormal 'lumps and bumps' (Figure 8.14). Repeating the tracing using a different lead (V1, MCL1 or III) can also help to identify missing P waves.

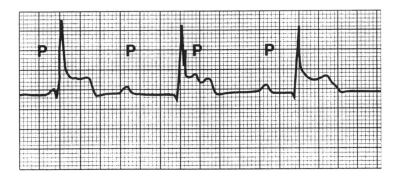

Figure 8.14 P waves hidden in the QRS complex

Occasionally, hidden P waves can be revealed by slowing the ventricular rate by vagal stimulation from carotid sinus massage or drugs.

Abnormally shaped P ('ectopic') waves indicate that the direction of depolarization through the atria is abnormal and consequently has not been initiated by the SAN. They have two possible sources:

- Premature beats.

- Escape beats.

Premature beats
As these usually originate in the atria and, rarely, from the atrioventricular junction they are known as **atrial** and **junctional premature beats**, respectively.

A distinguishing feature of a premature beat is the coupling interval, i.e. the time between the normal P wave and the abnormal one (P'). This is shorter than that between two normal P waves (PP) because the myocardial focus, giving rise to the premature atrial beat, depolarizes before the SAN (Figure 8.15). The coupling interval is constant if the premature beat is always produced from the same focus.

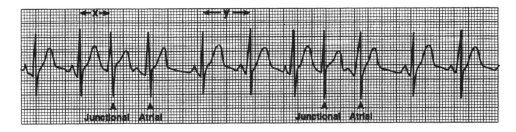

Figure 8.15 Ectopic P waves.

The premature P wave (P') (Figure 8.15) blocks the SAN from discharging and so disturbs the subsequent rhythm of P wave production. This can be demonstrated on the rhythm strip by noting the interval between the normal P waves on either side of the ectopic beat. This distance is less than twice the normal PP interval.

The focus may produce single or multiple premature beats. A tachycardia is defined as having three or more such beats occurring in rapid succession. If they occur in discrete self-terminating runs, they are described as being **paroxysmal**. When they occur in longer runs, the abnormal focus may take over completely and not allow any normal (SAN-generated) P waves to occur for a prolonged period of time. In these cases it is important to study the whole rhythm strip to determine if a normal PP interval can be found.

Escape beats

If the SAN fails to send out its electrical impulse another part of the conduction system will discharge instead. This gives rise to an escape beat (Figure 8.16). As it occurs later than expected, the coupling interval between the normal and escape P wave is longer than the normal (SAN-generated) PP interval.

Premature beat: Reduced coupling interval
Escape beat: Increased coupling interval

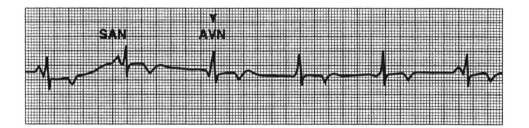

**Figure 8.16
Escape P waves**

Is there atrial flutter?

In this condition the atria are depolarizing at 250–350 beats/min but in most cases the rate is very close to 300 beats/min (i.e. one per big square). This atrial activity gives rise to regular F waves. When runs of these waves occur the baseline develops a characteristic 'sawtooth' appearance (Figure 8.17).

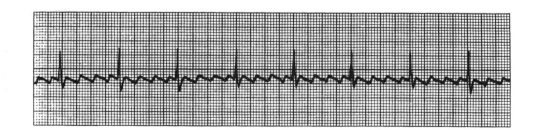

**Figure 8.17
Atrial flutter**

Only rarely does the AVN conduct all the atrial impulses to the ventricles. More commonly only one in two or one in four get through. Nevertheless, the QRS complexes which result have a normal shape if the remaining part of the conduction system has not been altered. If the diagnosis is in doubt, carotid sinus massage can be used to temporarily increase the degree of AVN block so that F waves can be seen.

Are the number of P and QRS waves the same?

If the number of P and QRS waves are the same, measure the PR interval. In first-degree heart block the number of P waves is the same as the number of QRS complexes but the PR interval is constant and longer than 0.2 s (one large square) (Figure 8.18). This condition is an ECG diagnosis and generally does not progress to more serious forms of heart block. It can, however, result from digitalis, beta-blockers and rheumatic myocarditis.

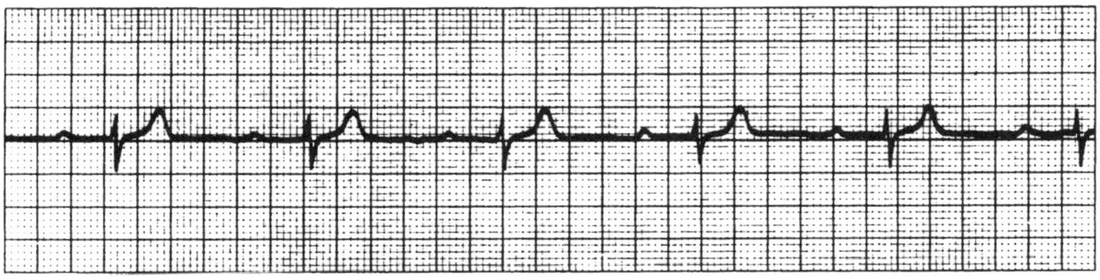

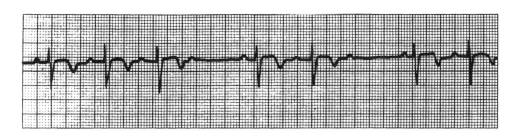

**Figure 8.18
First-degree
block**

If there are more P waves than QRS complexes then the patient has either second- or third-degree heart block. To distinguish between them the PR interval must be examined.

Second-degree heart block – Mobitz type I (Wenckebach)
In this condition the PR interval progressively lengthens until a P wave is not followed by a QRS complex. The AVN then recovers and the next PR interval reverts to the previous shortest conduction time. This rhythm is therefore distinguished by having both varying PR and RR intervals (Figure 8.19). In some cases this phenomenon is physiological; in others it can be the result of inferior myocardial infarction, digitalis or rheumatic myocarditis.

**Figure 8.19
Second-degree
block – Mobitz
type I**

Second-degree heart block – Mobitz type II

In this condition there is an intermittent non-conduction of some P waves but the PR interval remains constant (Figure 8.20). However, it may be of a normal or prolonged duration. Mobitz type II is much more likely to progress to third-degree heart block than type I and there is a higher chance of developing asystole or ventricular dysrhythmias (see later).

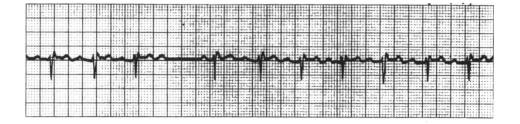

Figure 8.20 Second-degree block – Mobitz type II

Third-degree (complete) heart block

This results in total dissociation between the depolarization of the atria and ventricles with each beating independently (Figure 8.21). As a consequence, there is no consistent relationship between P waves and the QRS complexes on the ECG trace. The PR interval is therefore completely erratic but the PP and RR intervals are constant.

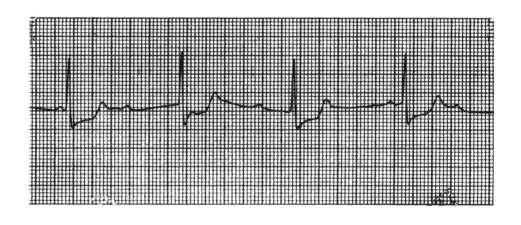

Figure 8.21 Third-degree (complete) block

The QRS complex can be narrow or wide depending on the source of the ventricular pacemaker. A focus near the AVN will result in a rate of around 50/min with narrow complexes as they are conducted via the bundle of His. This can result from congenital abnormalities but is also associated with inferior myocardial infarction.

A ventricular focus more distal from the AVN will produce a rate of around 30/min. However the QRS complexes will be wide (over 0.10 s) because conduction through the ventricles is not by the normal pathway. This can result from congenital abnormalities as well as from anterior and inferior myocardial infarction. These patients have a worse prognosis than those with a narrow QRS.

Table 8.1

Block	P:QRS	PR interval	RR interval
First-degree	Equal	Constant and prolonged	Constant
Second-degree, type I	P > QRS	Variable	Variable
Second-degree, type II	P > QRS	Constant	Variable
Third-degree	P > QRS	Variable	Constant

Is the QRS duration normal?

The normal duration for the QRS is 0.10 s (2.5 little squares) or less. This can occur only if the ventricular depolarization originates from above the bifurcation of the bundle of His. Broader complexes occur as a result of:

- Ventricular premature beats.

- Ventricular escape beats.

- Bundle branch blocks.

- Left ventricular hypertrophy.

Ventricular premature beats (VPB)
These present as bizarre, wide complexes with abnormal ST and T waves (Figure 8.22). Unlike the normal situation, ventricular depolarization is premature, thereby reducing the interval between the normal and abnormal beats (RR').

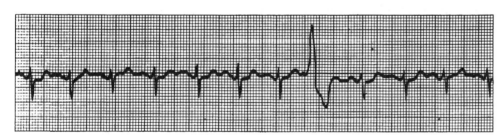

Figure 8.22 Ventricular ectopic

In contrast to the atrial premature beats, ventricular premature beats do not alter, or reset, the SAN. Consequently, the frequency of the P waves will continue undisturbed by the abnormal ventricular activity. There is therefore usually a compensatory pause after the ventricular premature beat and the following P wave occurs at the normal time.

A ventricular premature beat discharging during the repolarization phase of the ventricle runs the risk of precipitating ventricular fibrillation. The chances of this are thought to be higher if the beat occurs close to the T wave. This is known as the **R-on-T phenomenon** (Figure 8.23).

Figure 8.23 R-on-T ectopic

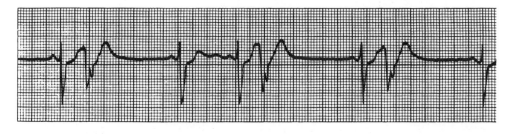

When there is more than one ventricular premature beat, specific terms are used if other features exist:

- **Multifocal ventricular ectopics**: when the VPB varies in shape from beat to beat (Figure 8.24). This may or may not represent a number of separate foci but it does indicate a significant increase in ventricular excitability and a higher chance of deteriorating into ventricular fibrillation.

Figure 8.24 Multifocal ventricular ectopics

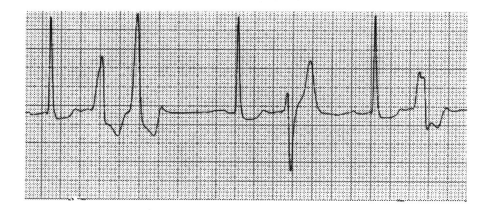

- **Bigemini**: when a normal QRS complex is followed by a ventricular premature beat (Figure 8.25).

Figure 8.25 Bigemini

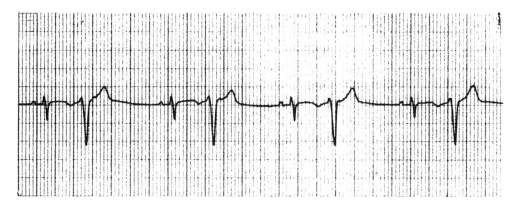
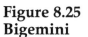

- **Trigemini**: when two normal consecutive QRS complexes are followed by a ventricular premature beat (Figure 8.26).

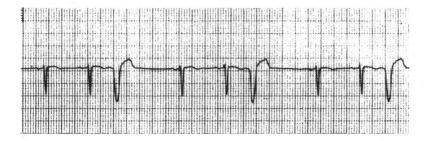

Figure 8.26
Trigemini

- **Couplet**: when there are two ventricular ectopic beats in a row (Figure 8.27).

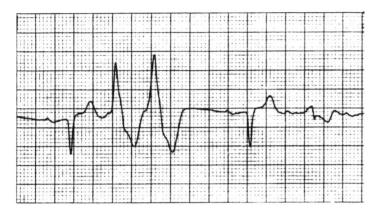

Figure 8.27
Couplets

Ventricular escape beats

These occur when the SAN and AVN can no longer generate an electrical impulse or stimulate the ventricles. In such circumstances the ventricles have to rely upon their own intrinsic pacemaker (see earlier in this chapter). Consequently the heart rate is slow and the RR' interval is longer than normal. If P waves exist they do not have any connection to the QRS (see Third-degree heart block, page 116).

Aberrant conduction with supraventricular premature stimulation

The QRS is abnormal because the premature atrial impulse gets to either the AVN or the ventricles before they have had a chance to repolarize fully from the preceding stimulation. Consequently, the conduction through the ventricles is abnormal and the resulting QRS complex is broad and abnormal in shape. Occasionally the shape of the QRS varies from beat to beat because the conduction pathway through the ventricles is not consistent. The PR interval is normal or slightly prolonged in this condition.

Is there ventricular tachycardia?

This occurs when there are three or more consecutive ventricular premature beats, with a rate greater than 140/min. It is said to be sustained if it lasts more than 30 s (Figure 8.28).

**Figure 8.28
Ventricular
tachycardia**

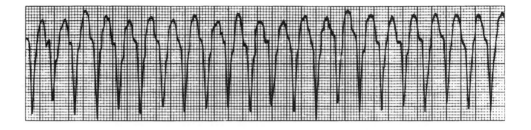

Ventricular tachycardia produces a regular, or almost regular, rhythm with a constantly abnormally wide QRS complex. The rate usually lies between 140 and 280 beats/min.

A regular, broad QRS complex tachycardia can also be due to a supraventricular rhythm with an aberrant conduction. Occasionally the abnormal QRS complexes existed before the SVT started and the increase in rate simply reflects the increase in rate of stimulation from the atria. However, the complexes may become abnormal only once the SVT starts. In these circumstances the conducting system cannot repolarize quickly enough for the new wave of depolarization from the atria. As a consequence the ventricular depolarization takes an abnormal route and this is reflected in the abnormal QRS shape.

Distinguishing between VT and SVT with aberrant conduction can be difficult. A search must therefore be made for the following features.

Fusion beats are produced when the atrial electrical impulse partially depolarizes the ventricular muscle which has not been fully depolarized by the ventricular premature beat.

Capture beats occur in the context of atrioventricular dissociation, when the atrial electrical impulse completely depolarises the ventricle before it is depolarized by the ventricular premature beat. The effect is a normal QRS complex in the midst of the sequence of broad QRS complexes.

If the QRS complex was broad before the tachycardia started, and its shape did not change after the tachycardia commenced, then the dysrhythmia is likely to be an SVT with aberrant conduction. It follows that access to previous ECG recordings is required before this can be determined.

Further clues as to the origin of the broad complex tachycardia come from studying the patient's 12-lead ECG, previous ECG tracings and medical notes. It is therefore essential that attempts are made to obtain these records. However, even after careful ECG evaluation it may still be impossible to distinguish between VT and a supraventricular rhythm with an aberrant conduction. In these cases, and especially after myocardial infarction, it is always safer to assume a ventricular origin for a broad complex tachycardia.

Table 8.2 Ventricular tachycardia vs SVT with aberrant conduction

	VT	SVT and aberrant conduction
Fusion beats	Yes	No
Capture beats	Yes	No
P waves	Absent or not connected with the QRS	Precede QRS

Is there Torsade de pointes?

This is a type of ventricular tachycardia where the cardiac axis is constantly changing in a regular fashion (Figure 8.29).

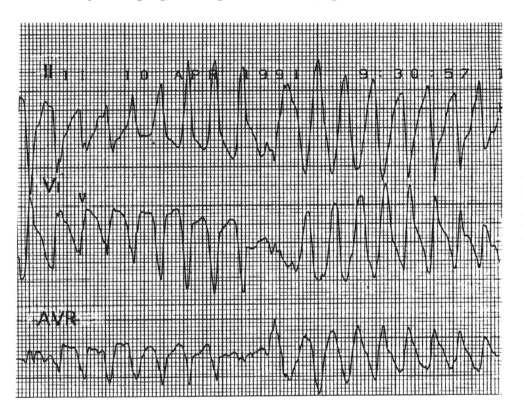
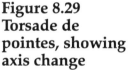

Figure 8.29 Torsade de pointes, showing axis change

Although it can occur spontaneously, it can also result from ischaemic heart disease, hypokalaemia and certain drugs which increase the QT interval (examples are tricyclic antidepressants (see Chapter 13) and the class 1a anti-arrhythmic agents (see Chapter 3)). This condition can end spontaneously or degenerate into VF. Interestingly, VF may have a similar pattern, particularly shortly after its onset, but this is usually short lived. Continued observation of the ECG will reveal a far more random appearance and greater variability in QRS morphology in the case of VF.

Atrial fibrillation in the presence of an anomalous conducting pathway that bypasses the AVN may permit rapid transmission of atrial impulses to the ventricles. The resulting ventricular rate may be so fast that cardiac output falls dramatically. The ECG appearances are of a very rapid, broad complex tachycardia that may show marked variability in the QRS complexes. However, the QRS complexes do not show the twisting axis characteristic of torsade de pointes. Furthermore, it is possible to recognize occasional fusion beats in cases of atrial fibrillation. The rhythm overall is also more organized than VF and lacks the random change in amplitude.

Is there an idioventricular rhythm (IVR)?

This occurs when the ventricles have taken over as the cardiac pacemaker due to failure of the SAN, atria or AVN. In view of the ventricle's slow intrinsic rate of depolarization the heart rate is usually slow (<40 beats/min). However, it can be accelerated and produce rates up to 120 beats/min.

Acute idioventricular rhythm commonly occurs after a myocardial infarction.

An **agonal rhythm** is characterized by the presence of slow, irregular, wide ventricular complexes of varying morphology. This rhythm is usually seen during the latter stages of unsuccessful resuscitation. The complexes gradually slow and often become progressively broader before all recognizable electrical actively is lost.

SUMMARY

The electrical activity of the heart is highly organized and monitoring of this activity should be carried out in a particular way to minimize the chances of artefacts. By using a systematic approach it is possible to interpret ECG rhythm strips effectively.

It is important to remember that it is the patient, and not the monitor, which should be treated.

——— 9 ———
Treatment protocols

Objectives

After reading this chapter you should be able to:

- Understand the order of treatments in cardiac arrest rhythms
- Understand the order of treatments in bradyarrhythmias
- Understand the order of treatments in tachyarrhyhmias

INTRODUCTION

This chapter deals with the nature and order of electrical and pharmacological treatments for various dysrhythmias.

In order to apply the protocols correctly the advanced life support (ALS) provider must be proficient at dysrhythmia recognition and have a thorough knowledge of the defibrillator and drugs used. However, the protocols cannot be applied safely without first diagnosing cardiac arrest and establishing effective basic life support (BLS), and then diagnosing the dysrhythmia involved. This approach must be used so that the crucial step of starting BLS is not delayed. Rhythm recognition and the commencement of BLS may occur simultaneously during a team approach to cardiac arrest. This is particularly important when diagnosing ventricular fibrillation as the time taken to deliver the first shock is critical in determining outcome.

The protocols are presented as algorithms in two groups:

1. **Cardiac arrest rhythms**: ventricular fibrillation (VF)/pulseless ventricular tachycardia, (VT) and non-VF/VT (asystole, electromechanical dissociation (EMD)).
2. **Peri-arrest rhythms:** bradyarrhythmias, tachyarrhythmias: broad complex tachycardia, narrow complex tachycardia (SVT).

Paediatric protocols are shown in Chapter 12.

Always remember: treat the patient not the monitor

CARDIAC ARREST RHYTHMS

The 1997 resuscitation guidelines for use in the UK use a single universal algorithm for the management of cardiac arrest (Figure 9.1).

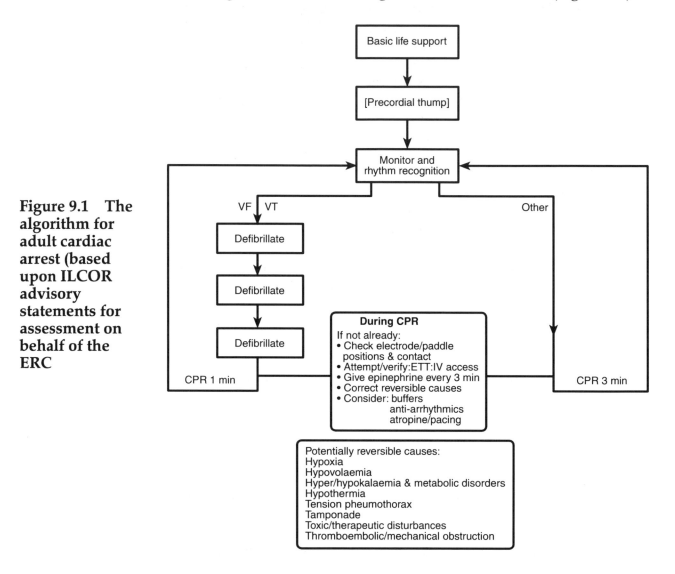

Figure 9.1 The algorithm for adult cardiac arrest (based upon ILCOR advisory statements for assessment on behalf of the ERC

Ventricular fibrillation/pulseless ventricular tachycardia

Emphasis is now placed on the identification and treatment of ventricular fibrillation as this is the most common arrest arrhythmia and the one from which the largest group of survivors comes. It may be preceded by a period of pulseless ventricular tachycardia. The treatment of both conditions is the same – defibrillation – and the time to delivery of the first shock is critical, as conditions for an optimal outcome may exist for as little as 90 s. Therefore defibrillation is the first manoeuvre to be performed in ALS. The only exception to this is when the cardiac arrest was witnessed or monitored and defibrillation is preceded by a precordial thump. This is a sharp blow, delivered to the patient's sternum with a closed fist, which delivers a small amount of mechanical energy to the myocardium.

If performed early enough after the onset of VF it may convert the rhythm to one which restores the circulation.

The ECG monitor should be attached without delay and in the presence of VF/pulseless VT, three shocks using energies of 200 J, 200 J, 360 J, are delivered in quick succession (30–45 s). The paddles are left in position while the defibrillator is recharged and the monitor is observed for rhythm changes. The carotid pulse is palpated for evidence of a circulation for 5 s (usually by the team member who is managing the airway) only if after defibrillation the rhythm changes to one normally capable of sustaining a circulation. This method optimizes defibrillation, as each shock lowers the chest impedance, increasing the energy delivered to the heart by subsequent shocks. Clearly if the rhythm changes at any time not all three shocks will be required.

The practical skill of defibrillation is dealt with in Chapter 16, but several points must be remembered: it is vital to remember team safety when delivering a rapid sequence of shocks – always ensure that everybody is clear from the patient before defibrillating, that GTN patches have been removed before defibrillating, avoid placing paddles close to pacemakers and use conductive gel or gel pads which must be replaced after three loops have been completed.

If these initial shocks are unsuccessful, CPR is instituted for 1 min, during which time intubation and/or intravenous access are attempted and adrenaline (epinephrine) administered, 1 mg IV or 2–3 mg intratracheal. When the tracheal route is used, the drug should be diluted to 10 ml and administration followed by 5 ventilations to aid dispersion and absorption. This loop is now repeated, this time with three shocks, each at 360 J, with the monitor being checked between each one.

The interval between the third and fourth shocks must be not longer than 1 min

CPR is continued for a further 1 min, during which further attempts are made at advanced airway techniques and venous access. If there are sufficient members in a cardiac arrest team intubation and cannulation may be performed concurrently, but this must not be at the expense of delaying CPR or defibrillation.

1 mg adrenaline should be given intravenously every 3 min during the resuscitation of a patient who has suffered a cardiac arrest

Where VF is refractory to treatment, the use of sodium bicarbonate can be considered along with other anti-arrhythmic agents such as lignocaine or Bretylium. Also, consider changing the paddle position to anteroposterior, trying a different defibrillator and consider

125

other reversible causes. The most common reason for failure to defribrillate is poor paddle or electrode application.

These loops are continued until the patient is resuscitated or the team leader, in discussion with the team, decides to stop resuscitation.

If during application of the VF protocol defibrillation leads to a change of rhythm and restoration of a cardiac output, which subsequently reverts to VF, the protocol must be reapplied from the beginning, i.e. from the first 200 J shock, otherwise the shock energy remains at 360 J.

Synchronized defibrillation

In VF a DC shock is delivered at random, i.e. unsynchronized. When attempting to cardiovert VT the shock is best delivered co-ordinated with the R wave, i.e. synchronized and the defibrillator must be set accordingly. If the shock is delivered on the T wave, when the heart is refractory, then VF may be precipitated (see Chapter 16).

Non-VF, non-pulseless VT

In these circumstances it is essential to exclude the possibility of VF/VT, after which the right-hand side of the algorithm in Figure 9.1 is followed.

Asystole

The outcome from asystole is poor unless there are still P waves present and it is therefore essential to ensure that the correct diagnosis has been made, most importantly to avoid misdiagnosis of fine VF. This may be due to misinterpretation because it is very fine or due to equipment failure, for example disconnection of an ECG lead or setting the gain too low. If any doubt exists, treatment begins as for VF with three shocks in rapid succession. The risks of not treating VF are greater than those of three unnecessary shocks. Similarly, a precordial thump can be used under the same criteria as for VF.

As soon as asystole is diagnosed, or immediately after three shocks, CPR should be started (or recommenced), during which the patient should be intubated or intravenous access obtained and the first dose of adrenaline given. Atropine should also be given, in a single dose of 3 mg IV or 6 mg intratracheal, the aim being to achieve complete block of the vagus.

The ECG should now be carefully checked for the presence of P waves or slow ventricular activity. If either of these are present then transvenous or external pacing should be considered. If there is no electrical activity, CPR should be continued and further doses of adrenaline administered every 3 min. After 3 loops a single dose of 5 mg of adrenaline can also be tried. Unfortunately, the outcome from asystole after 15–20 min of resuscitation is very poor.

If, during application of this protocol, asystole changes to another rhythm which subsequently reverts to asystole, the protocol should be reapplied from the beginning. However, if 3 mg atropine has already been given in the initial loop, the dose should not be repeated.

Electromechanical dissociation

The outcome from EMD is poor unless there is a secondary cause for it. If one is found and treated promptly the outlook dramatically improves. The main aim in managing a patient in EMD is to rapidly assess whether a treatable cause exists, and to treat it promptly and effectively. Treatable causes fall into two main groups, the 4 H's and 4 T's which are listed in the algorithm in Figure 9.1.

The patient in EMD should be managed using the right-hand side of the algorithm in Figure 9.1. CPR is started, during which intubation and intravenous access are attempted. Adrenaline is given in the appropriate dose and repeated every 3 min, while potentially reversible causes are sought.

Resuscitation must not be withheld while these conditions are sought; they must be eliminated or treated appropriately while resuscitation is in progress

Potentially reversible causes – the 4 H's and 4 T's

Hypoxia

Every attempt should be made to secure the airway, preferably by inserting a cuffed tracheal tube. If this is not possible one of the alternatives described in Chapter 6 should be used. All patients should be ventilated with 100% oxygen. The most common cause of persistent hypoxia is unrecognized misplacement of an advanced airway device.

Hypovolaemia

Hypovolaemia of such a degree that it causes EMD is usually due to bleeding. Trauma, with its attendant problems, is a common cause in all age groups. Other sources not seen infrequently include ruptured aortic aneurysm and massive gastrointestinal bleeding. Hypovolaemia should always be considered in children: this is dealt with in Chapter 12.

Treatment consists of rapid replacement of the intravascular volume with appropriate fluids and surgery where necessary to stop haemorrhage wherever possible.

External cardiac massage is less effective in the hypovolaemic patient and, if suitably skilled help is available, thoracotomy and internal cardiac massage should be considered. It must be emphasized that thoracotomy is only a temporizing measure, and should be performed only if immediate treatment of the underlying cause of hypovolaemia can be undertaken.

Hyperkalaemia/hypocalcaemia and metabolic disorders

Hyperkalaemia and hypocalcaemia may be known to exist from previous tests, but are frequently discovered biochemically only after the resuscitation has failed. Nevertheless some common biochemical abnormality can be predicted from the history. For instance, chronic diuretic usage may be associated with hypokalaemia, while a patient in end-stage renal disease who is dependent on haemodialysis, is likely to be hyperkalaemic or hypocalcaemic. Acute pancreatitis and, more rarely, hydrofluoric acid burns can also cause hypocalcaemia. Burns and severe crush injury can both result in hyperkalaemia.

ECG changes may occasionally be diagnostic, as shown in Table 9.1.

Table 9.1   ECG changes

	Hyperkalaemia	Hypocalcaemia
P	Flattened	N
QRS	Widened	N
QT	N	Prolonged
T	Peaked	N

The use of calcium chloride in EMD has been restricted to treatment of hyperkalaemia and hypocalcaemia.

Hypothermia is covered in Chapter 13.

Tension pneumothorax

This may be either the primary cause of the arrest or secondary to therapeutic manoeuvres (especially central venous line placement). The diagnosis is clinical and is made by searching for the following signs:

- Unilateral absence of breath sounds.
- Unilateral hyperresonant percussion note.
- Tracheal deviation.

Once the diagnosis has been made the chest should be rapidly decompressed – initially by needle thoracocentesis and then by chest drain placement (see Chapter 16).

Time should not be wasted taking a chest radiograph if this diagnosis is suspected.

Tamponade

This is a difficult diagnosis during cardiac arrest, and a high index of suspicion is necessary if it is to be made. The history may occasionally be diagnostic (for instance a stab wound over the precordium); examination is rarely helpful as all the signs of Beck's triad (venous pressure elevation, muffled heart sounds and decline in arterial pressure with inspiration) are obscured by the arrest itself. Thus, if other treatable causes of EMD have been eliminated, and a satisfactory output cannot be obtained with external cardiac massage, needle pericardiocentesis should be performed (see Chapter 16).

Toxic/therapeutic disturbances

Many patients with ischaemic heart disease are on calcium antagonists, and this information should be actively sought during resuscitation. Poisoning is covered in Chapter 13.

Thromboembolic/mechanical obstruction

The diagnosis of pulmonary embolism can be made only on the history. There is no simple treatment, but it is said that vigorous external cardiac massage may occasionally dislodge the clot. In centres that have the facilities immediate cardiopulmonary bypass followed by operative removal of the clot is life saving.

PERI-ARREST RHYTHMS

Before, or immediately after, a cardiac arrest a patient may exhibit a variety of arrhythmias. The following section provides details of how to manage three of the most common arrhythmias, based upon the recommendations of the European Resuscitation Council (1996). After initial assessment and treatment emphasis is placed upon calling for expert help. In recognition of the fact that this is not always immediately available, information is provided on the most appropriate management. It must be stressed, however, that these algorithms cannot cover all the possible arrhythmias which may occur in the peri-arrest period, nor indeed can every possible variation in treatment be included. There are two final 'rules' which must be remembered when treating arrhythmias:

1. Always treat the patient, not the monitor
2. Any intervention to treat an arrhythmia, e.g. drugs or electricity, can also cause an arrhythmia.

In all situations, it is assumed that oxygen is already being administered and venous access has been secured

Bradyarrhythmias

These are due to either a bradycardia or the presence of heart block. Although a bradycardia has been defined as a ventricular rate of <60/min, not all patients with a heart rate of <60/min will require treatment, the deciding factors being the patient's haemodynamic state. Conversely, in a patient with a low cardiac output a rate of 70/min may be inadequate. Furthermore, complete heart block with narrow QRS complexes is not an immediate indication for treatment, as this is often associated with a stable rhythm and an adequate cardiac output.

Therefore, in the decision to treat bradyarrhythmias, two questions must be answered:

- Does the rhythm have the potential to cause asystole?

- Does the patient exhibit signs or symptoms that suggest that treatment is needed?

The complete algorithm is shown in Figure 9.2.

A risk of asystole exists:

- With a history of asystole.

- When there is any pause of ⩾ 3 s or more.

- In the presence of Mobitz type II heart block or complete heart block with wide QRS complexes.

If any of these exist initial treatment is with atropine 500 μg IV (repeated to a maximum of 3 mg), then **expert help must be sought**.

Significant signs and symptoms are:

- Low cardiac output: congestive cardiac failure, dyspnoea, altered mental state.

- Hypotension, systolic blood pressure ⩽ 90 mmHg.

- Heart rate < 40/min.

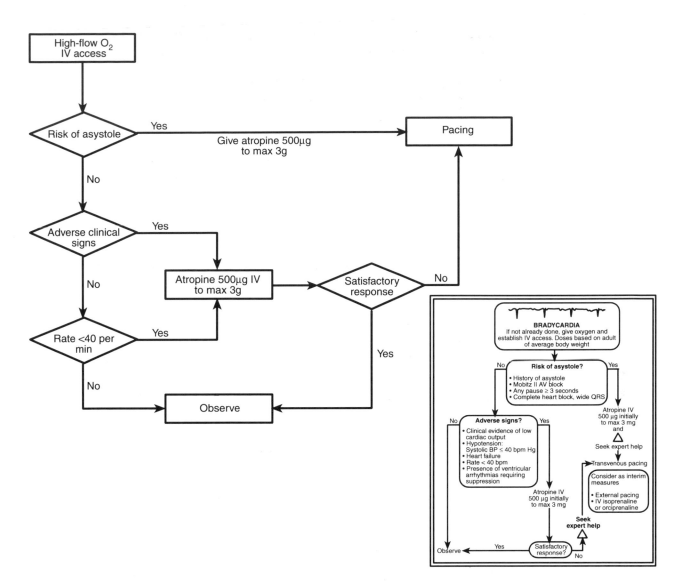

Figure 9.2 **Algorithm for bradycardia. Inset shows the original ERC algorithm**

In addition, against a background bradycardia a ventricular tachy-arrhythmia which requires suppression may emerge.

If any of these exist, initial treatment is with atropine 500 µg IV (repeated to a maximum of 3 mg), then **expert help must be sought**.

Further (expert) management will consist of increasing the patient's heart rate by pacing. The insertion of a transvenous pacing wire will require specific skills and takes time. If this is not immediately accessible, alternatives are external pacing or the use of an isoprenaline infusion, starting initially at a rate of 1 µg/min (via a central line). This rate may have to be increased but remember the risk of precipitating further arrhythmias.

Broad complex tachycardia

When faced with a broad complex tachycardia (QRS >0.1 s), the safest course of action is to assume that it is ventricular in origin and treat it accordingly. (Although technically it might be supraventricular with aberrant conduction, little harm results treating it as ventricular, whereas the converse is not safe.) The complete algorithm is shown in Figure 9.3.

The first step is to rapidly establish whether the patient has a palpable pulse. If not, then the patient should be managed according

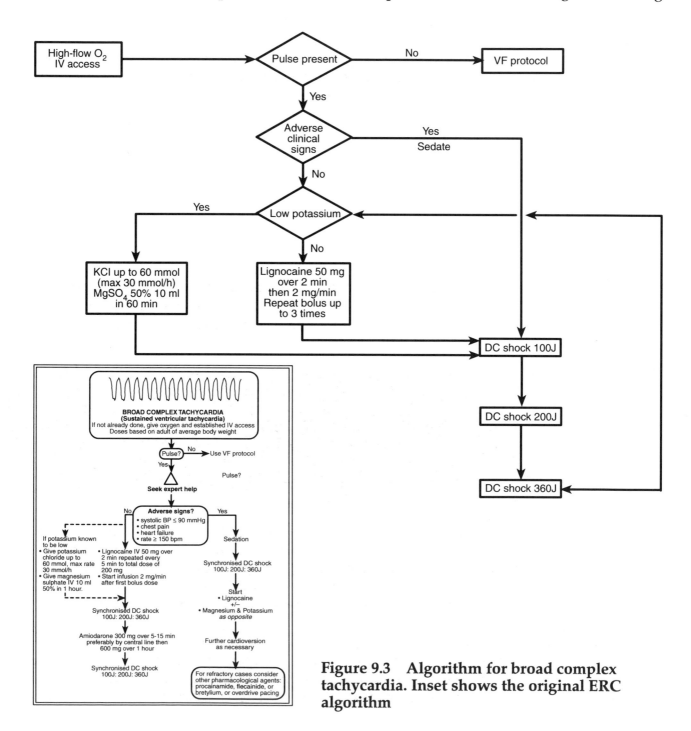

Figure 9.3 Algorithm for broad complex tachycardia. Inset shows the original ERC algorithm

to the guidelines for pulseless ventricular tachycardia already described.

If the patient does have a pulse, do they have any of the following adverse signs or symptoms?

- Hypotension, systolic blood pressure $\leq$ 90 mmHg.
- Heart rate $\geq$ 150/min.
- Chest pain.
- Low cardiac output: dyspnoea, heart failure, altered mental state.

If any of these are present, **seek expert help**. Emergency cardioversion is the treatment of choice, using a synchronized DC shock. If this is unsuccessful, lignocaine, magnesium and potassium (to ensure serum K^+ >3.6 mmol/l) should be administered followed by further attempts at cardioversion.

The initial management of the asymptomatic patient consists of correcting any hypokalaemia, administering magnesium and lignocaine. Once this is under way, **seek expert help**. If this treatment is ineffective, synchronized cardioversion may be required. If, however, the patient remains asymptomatic, amiodarone may be used.

Narrow complex tachycardia

Most often an SVT, narrow complex tachycardia is less frequent and less hazardous to patients than a ventricular tachycardia. Occasionally the arrhythmia may be atrial fibrillation which, at fast rates, may be difficult to diagnose. The complete algorithm for treatment is shown in Figure 9.4.

Initial treatment of a narrow complex tachycardia consists of stimulating the vagus nerve to try to reduce the rate. This can be achieved either by carotid sinus massage or by getting the patient to perform a Valsalva manoeuvre (forced expiration against a closed glottis). It must be borne in mind that the former may rupture a plaque within the carotid artery which, if it embolizes, may cause the patient to suffer a cerebrovascular accident. Profound vagal stimulation can also cause a severe bradycardia, which may trigger ventricular fibrillation in the acute ischaemic state or in the presence of digitalis toxicity.

If these manoeuvres are unsuccessful, then the treatment of choice is a rapid intravenous bolus (3 mg) of adenosine. This can be increased in steps to a maximum of two injections each of 12 mg. If adenosine is administered, it is important to warn the patient of brief but unpleasant side effects, including flushing, nausea and

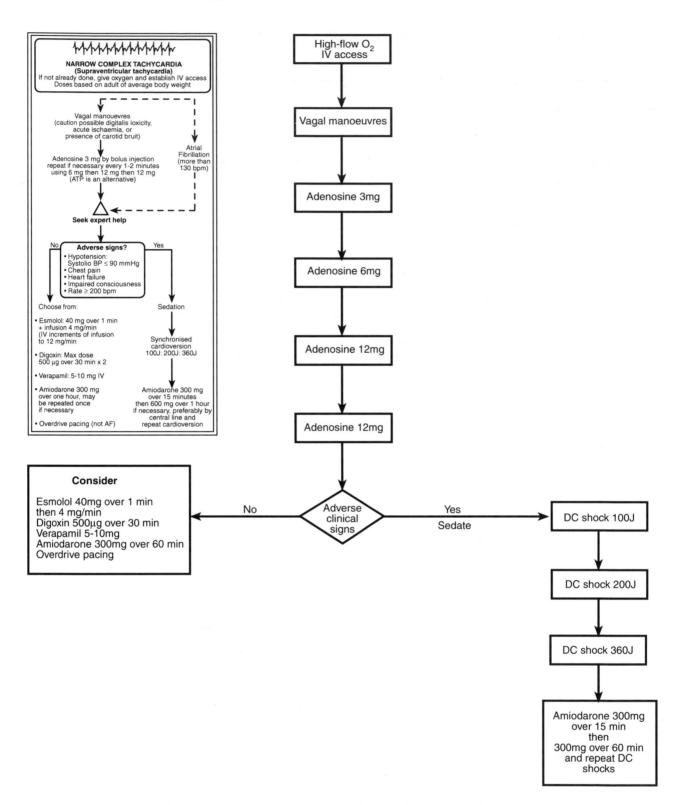

Figure 9.4 Algorithm for narrow complex tachycardia. Inset shows the original ERC algorithm

chest discomfort. If adenosine fails or a diagnosis of atrial fibrillation at a rate >130/min is made, then **seek expert help**.

134

Next, assess the patient for the presence of adverse signs or symptoms:

- Hypotension, systolic blood pressure ≤ 90 mmHg.
- Heart rate ≥ 200/min.
- Chest pain.
- Low cardiac output: congestive cardiac failure, altered mental state, dyspnoea.

If adverse signs are present, treatment is by synchronized cardioversion with a DC shock. This may need to be repeated if unsuccessful after the administration of amiodarone.

In the patient who remains asymptomatic, a variety of pharmacological treatments, including esmolol (a very short acting beta-blocker), digoxin or amiodarone, may be tried. Although verapamil is widely used in these circumstances, it must not be used in conjunction with intravenous beta-blockers because of the risk of precipitating asystole. In highly specialized units, overdrive pacing is another alternative.

Cardioversion

The delivery of a DC shock, or cardioversion, is used in the management of both ventricular and supraventricular tachycardias. Unlike the management of ventricular fibrillation, it is important that the energy is delivered at the correct point in the ECG – synchronized with the R wave (hence 'synchronized' cardioversion). If the shock is delivered to coincide with the T wave, during the refractory period, ventricular fibrillation may be precipitated. Because the defibrillator paddles are used as the electrodes to monitor the rhythm, they must be kept well applied to the chest wall to reduce artefact or loss of signal, which will delay the delivery of the shock. Occasionally, in the symptomatic patient with very fast ventricular tachycardia, it may prove difficult to distinguish QRS and T waves. If the delays are excessive then an unsynchronized shock should be used.

——10——
Post-resuscitation care

Objectives

After reading this chapter you should be able to:

- Understand the spectrum of outcomes after resuscitation
- Understand the spectrum of care that may be needed
- Understand the approach to patient assessment
- Understand the initiation of the diagnostic work-up
- Understand the basics of CCU and ICU treatment
- Understand the pointers to likely neurological outcome

SPECTRUM OF OUTCOMES

The aim of resuscitation is to produce a fully conscious, neurologically intact patient who has a spontaneous and stable cardiac rhythm with adequate cardiorespiratory function. The return of a spontaneous circulation alone does not indicate the end of a successful resuscitation: more probably, it marks the start of a long and difficult post-resuscitation care phase.

The patient may recover almost immediately following early and effective resuscitation after primary cardiac arrest. If stable, these patients can usually be transferred to a coronary care unit (CCU) for observation.

Occasionally, resuscitation is more prolonged and the patient's level of consciousness depressed. Mechanical ventilation may be needed due to inadequate spontaneous respiration and drug therapy is required to maintain the circulation. These patients will require transfer to an intensive care unit (ICU) for assisted ventilation and haemodynamic monitoring, once they are stable enough to be moved safely. Not all patients will fit into one of these situations and a whole spectrum of outcomes exist between these two extremes. Ultimately care will depend upon local expertise and facilities available.

INITIAL ASSESSMENT

History before transfer

A careful evaluation should be obtained prior to transfer, including any antecedent history. In hospital, if the patient is found to have an end-stage or terminal condition it may be deemed correct to leave the patient on the ward and to withhold further therapy, providing the correct protocols have been followed.

A history of overdose, especially of tricyclic antidepressants or narcotics, is an invaluable guide to specific therapy.

The possibility of hypoglycaemic or hypoxia-induced arrest must be ascertained, and consideration given to whether the cardiac arrest was preceded by a neurological event such as an intracerebral haemorrhage (stroke).

An estimate of the duration of arrest prior to starting resuscitation is prognostically important. The duration of CPR and drugs given should always be determined.

Examination and treatment before transfer

Before transfer, rapid examination of the patient will rule out easily correctable problems and establish a baseline.

Examine the respiratory system

Rule out a tension pneumothorax and confirm position of the endotracheal tube by listening for breath sounds and watching chest movements. If available monitor end tidal carbon dioxide. Commonly the endotracheal tube has been inserted too far (more than 22 cm on average) and usually enters the right main bronchus, reducing air entry on the left. Crepitus from fractured ribs may be apparent at this stage. A chest tube should be inserted if a needle thoracocentesis has been used to decompress a tension pneumothorax or in a patient with rib fractures who is being mechanically ventilated.

Examine the cardiovascular system

Listen for heart sounds and palpate the major pulses. Look at the neck veins. If they are grossly dilated, this may indicate acute right heart failure (pulmonary embolus), biventricular failure or cardiac tamponade. If the latter is diagnosed, then consideration should be given to needle aspiration (pericardiocentesis). Absence of neck veins may indicate severe hypovolaemia following haemorrhage, e.g. following trauma or ectopic pregnancy. If accompanied by absence of femoral but presence of brachial pulses, the possibility of an aortic aneurysm should be considered.

Look at the ECG monitor

Tall T waves are seen in the acute phase of myocardial infarction, or may indicate hyperkalaemia as a result of renal failure or crush injury. Treatment involves bolus doses of intravenous calcium (10–20 ml of 10% calcium gluconate) and a dextrose/insulin infusion. Arrhythmias following tricyclic poisoning need expert attention but consider hyperventilation, bicarbonate, magnesium and pacing.

Carry out a limited neurological assessment

Note the Glasgow Coma Scale score, pupil sizes, light and corneal reflexes. Look for obvious lateralizing signs: changes in limb tone or movement and reflexes. Narcotic overdose responds to intravenous naloxone and benzodiazepine overdose to flumazenil. Beware of provoking fits in mixed overdoses by injudicious use of flumazenil.

Examine the abdomen

This may detect a distended stomach or significant swellings such as aortic aneurysm. Obvious gastric dilatation should be decompressed by passage of a nasogastric tube and the bladder emptied by passage of a catheter.

CARE OF THE OPTIMALLY RESUSCITATED PATIENT

Oxygen should be given by facemask. A flow of 6 l/min gives an inspired concentration of 30–40% with a variable performance mask (e.g. MC mask). A Venturi mask delivers a fixed concentration of 24–60%, dependent on the mask chosen. Adequacy of oxygenation can be monitored initially using a pulse oximeter, providing the peripheral circulation is adequate. The best guide to oxygenation is analysis of an arterial blood sample. ECG monitoring must be instituted and intravenous access secured. Intravenous analgesia should be given (e.g. morphine 2 mg repeated as necessary), especially in myocardial infarction. Anti-arrhythmics such as lignocaine should be continued and the patient transferred to the CCU where further management of arrhythmias will be undertaken if needed and any further diagnostic work-up completed. The patient should be closely observed for any deterioration in organ function.

Thrombolytic agents are not contraindicated after a short period of CPR and should be administered as soon as possible after diagnosis of myocardial infarction. The appropriate agent for patients in whom invasive procedures are anticipated is rTPA.

CARE OF THE PATIENT REQUIRING ORGAN SUPPORT

Profound global ischaemia occurs during cardiac arrest and leads to rapid depletion of intracellular energy stores, depolarization of cell membranes, potassium loss and calcium influx. There is loss of cellular and organ function which paradoxically may worsen in the early recovery phase, the so-called 'reperfusion' injury.

From a practical point of view, intermittent positive pressure ventilation should be continued with 100% oxygen and ECG monitoring. Anti-arrhythmic and vasoactive therapies may be needed to stabilize the patient before and during transport to the ICU. In addition, sedative drugs and muscle relaxants are used to facilitate mechanical ventilation. At the ICU the diagnostic examination and investigations will be completed and treatments for organ support instituted.

Diagnostic work-up

Immediate investigations include a 12-lead ECG, chest radiograph and measurement of arterial blood gases, electrolytes, creatinine and blood sugar. A lactate measurement can give some estimate of the degree of tissue hypoxia. Central venous blood gases are measured if a central line has been inserted (see Chapter 4).

The chest radiograph is scrutinized for fractures. Broken ribs may often be visible on the straight chest film but if a fractured sternum is suspected a lateral film may be necessary for confirmation. Pneumothoraces are obvious if very large, but on supine films can be difficult to see, even by the experienced clinician. Parenchymal lung injury or aspiration are not uncommon during resuscitation. A large heart or widened mediastinum should be noted but cardiac tamponade is not always obvious. The position of the endotracheal tube, nasogastric tube and any intravascular lines or a pacing wire should be confirmed.

The 12-lead ECG is often necessary to distinguish ventricular from supraventricular arrhythmias, although in the immediate post-myocardial infarction period most are ventricular in origin (see Chapter 8). Changes may also be seen as a result of hyperkalaemia (tall T waves), pulmonary embolus with a right ventricular strain pattern (S wave lead I, Q wave and T wave inversion in lead III, rSR and T wave inversion in V_1) or of acute myocardial infarction (ST elevation, tall T waves).

Haemodynamic monitoring

Non-invasive and clinical assessments of cardiac function are inaccurate in at least 30–50% of patients admitted to intensive and coronary care units. Empirical therapy may be ineffectual or hazardous if a correct haemodynamic assessment has not been made.

Measurement of blood pressure

It is well known that in patients who are very vasoconstricted (have a high systemic vascular resistance) cuff blood pressure may be almost inaudible and peripheral pulses almost impalpable despite there being a normal central arterial pressure. Therefore a large artery such as the femoral or brachial may be cannulated for more accurate blood pressure recording.

Measurement of cardiac filling pressures and cardiac output

A central venous pressure line is useful for infusing vasoactive drugs and reflects right ventricular function in relation to venous return. It cannot be used reliably to estimate left ventricular function, nor is it a primary route for volume replacement.

Intense vasoconstriction may help to maintain a normal blood pressure, but this does not always mean there is an adequate cardiac output. It may therefore be necessary to use a pulmonary artery flotation catheter (Swan–Ganz catheter). This is a multilumen catheter, inserted via the central veins, through the right side of the heart to lie in the pulmonary artery. It allows measurement of the pulmonary artery pressure and cardiac output, and gives an indirect estimate of the pressure in the left atrium (the pulmonary artery occlusion or wedge pressure). These indices are used to judge the circulating volume and pumping ability of the heart. It also allows a more accurate mixed venous blood sample to be taken than from a CVP line.

Measurement of oxygen transport variables

Measurement and manipulation of oxygen transport variables is considered central to the rational treatment of these patients. By combining measurements of the oxygen content in arterial and mixed venous blood with the cardiac output it is possible to estimate the amount of oxygen transported to and consumed by the tissues. Shock is defined as a failure to deliver an adequate supply of oxygen and nutrients to the tissues, not simply a low blood pressure.

RESPIRATORY SUPPORT

The airway must be secure and adequate ventilation assured. In the majority of cases this will require endotracheal intubation and mechanical ventilation. The patient will need to be sedated and occasionally paralysed, to prevent him fighting the ventilator, which increases oxygen demand and impairs the efficiency of ventilation. Initially ventilation should be with 100% oxygen until arterial blood gases are measured. It may then be adjusted so that the Pa_{O_2} remains in the 12–5 kPa range. Continuous hyperventilation is not of major benefit and the Pa_{CO_2} can be kept in the 4–5 kPa range. If hypoxia persists, positive end expiratory pressure (PEEP) may be necessary, but it is essential to measure cardiac filling pressures and cardiac output before therapeutic PEEP is added since, although the Pa_{O_2} may improve, the cardiac output and hence oxygen delivery may fall.

CARDIOVASCULAR SUPPORT

Following myocardial infarction the following values are associated with improved outcome: cardiac index (cardiac output/body surface area) >2.2 l/min/m^2 with a pulmonary artery occlusion pressure <18 mmHg. Mean arterial pressure should preferably be near normal (80–100 mmHg) to maintain coronary artery perfusion pressure. Adequate tissue oxygenation is promoted by a mixed venous oxyhaemoglobin saturation (Sv$_{O_2}$) greater than 60%; however, paradoxically high values are seen in critically ill patients with impaired tissue oxygen uptake. Elevated plasma lactate levels help to distinguish this group. On the ICU, fluids and vasoconstrictors are often needed to improve circulatory function, although vasodilators, diuretics and inotropes are frequently also given to patients following myocardial infarction.

RENAL SUPPORT

Following a period of hypotension and hypoxia renal function is likely to suffer. Following catheterization urine volumes are measured hourly. An output of at least 0.5 ml/kg/h and preferably 1 ml/kg/h is the goal, because this reflects adequate organ perfusion. If mannitol or other diuretics have been used, their effects should be taken into consideration. Renal function is optimized by ensuring adequate cardiorespiratory status as described above. The administration of diuretics to an oliguric patient who is hypovolaemic, hypotensive and hypoxic is illogical. Although frusemide and mannitol may have a place in ensuring adequate tubular flow, the use of these agents has not been shown to reverse acute renal dysfunction if hypotension and tissue hypoxia persist.

NEUROLOGICAL SUPPORT

Cerebral perfusion pressure (CPP) is the difference between mean arterial pressure (MAP) and intracranial pressure (ICP):

$$CPP = MAP - ICP$$

Under normal circumstances CPP is approximately 80 mmHg, 60 mmHg being the lower limit of normal. It is important to maintain CPP at a normal or even high normal level in this group of patients. This is best achieved by minimizing known reasons for increased intracranial pressure such as hypercarbia, coughing or fighting the ventilator. The indiscriminate use of mannitol is not recommended unless intracranial pressure is being monitored. A normal or high normal MAP should be maintained, if this can be achieved without jeopardizing myocardial function. Cerebral blood flow is also enhanced by the maintenance of a low normal haematocrit. This 'hypervolaemic haemodilution' must be performed with concurrent use of a pulmonary artery catheter to avoid overloading the circulation and precipitating left ventricular failure. In all cases haemoconcentration is to be avoided by ensuring appropriate intravenous fluid replacement.

Patients who have sustained a hypoxic brain injury may develop 'cerebral oedema', causing a rise in ICP, thereby reducing cerebral perfusion. Appropriate therapy can be guided by monitoring ICP via an extradural or subdural pressure monitoring system. Recently interest has been shown in monitoring jugular venous oxygen saturation as an index of cerebral oxygenation.

Any increase in cerebral metabolism (e.g. fits, hyperpyrexia) should be treated promptly. Hyperglycaemia is harmful to ischaemic brain tissue and must be avoided.

Neurological outcome indicators

The brief neurological assessment carried out immediately post-resuscitation is of prognostic value although full neurological assessments are generally delayed until 6 and 24 h later to improve reproducibility.

143

Consciousness level is assessed by the Glasgow Coma Scale score (GCS):

Eye opening

1. Nil
2. To pain
3. To commands
4. Spontaneously

Motor response

1. Nil
2. Extension to pain
3. Abnormal flexion to pain
4. Withdraws to pain
5. Localizes to pain
6. Obeys commands

Verbal

1. Nil
2. Incomprehensible sounds
3. Inappropriate words
4. Confused
5. Orientated

Patients in coma have a GCS of 8 or less: they do not open their eyes, fail to obey commands and do not speak.

Hemisphere function is assessed by limb tone, power and reflexes to look for localizing signs.

Brain stem function is assessed by pupillary and corneal response, eye movements, cough and gag or grimace reflexes. The pupils are not useful immediately post-arrest as an indicator of cerebral dysfunction, because catecholamines and atropine are frequently given during CPR and can cause dilatation of the pupils.

It is important to rule out cerebral trauma, intoxication, severe sepsis or meningitis before making predictions of neurological outcome. The presence of seizures, which occur in approximately 25% of patients, is not of prognostic importance.

If CPR was initiated following a primary cardiac event, then the coma is of a hypoxic–ischaemic nature. Only 10–15% of patients remaining in coma for >6 h gain an independent existence and 20% will enter a persistent vegetative state.

By utilizing brain stem reflexes as well as the GCS one can be more certain of outcome. Absent brain stem reflexes almost precludes a good recovery, but not, of course, survival!

In the unsedated unparalysed patient a high (≥10) or low (3–4) GCS score at 48 h predicts outcome in 80% of cases.

GASTROINTESTINAL SUPPORT

The gut as an organ also suffers from the effects of low cardiac output and from reperfusion injury. Treatment is as above and aims to maintain the delivery of well oxygenated blood to all parts of the gut. Gastric dilatation should be prevented by the use of a nasogastric tube, and stress ulcer prophylaxis should be considered. Early enteric feeding is beneficial to gut function and reduces gastric erosions.

SUMMARY

The aims of resuscitating a patient who has suffered a cardiorespiratory arrest are to achieve stable and adequate cardiorespiratory function and full neurological recovery. In the immediate post-arrest period, some patients will not achieve this despite the best efforts of the cardiac arrest team, consequently varying degrees of physiological support will be required to optimize their outcome. This is best achieved by utilizing the information gained from invasive haemodynamic monitoring and the skills of the intensive care staff.

Nevertheless, care should be taken not to try to predict the outcome of the more obtunded patient immediately following return of their circulation by a cursory neurological examination.

11
Cardiopulmonary resuscitation – putting it all together

Objectives

After reading this chapter you should be able to:

- Understand the sequence of management in cardiopulmonary resuscitation
- Understand the roles within the resuscitation team
- Understand the role and responsibilities of the team leader

---

Although the initial aim in the management of any life-threatening emergency is to preserve life, the true measure of success is discharging a patient who is as well as, or better than, before. If a cardiac resuscitation attempt is to be successful to this degree, then correct management must start immediately, and must continue until the post-resuscitation care phase is finished. Failure to deliver optimum care at any stage will lessen the chances of a favourable outcome. There are no second chances.

The earlier chapters of this book have discussed the application of the knowledge and practical skills that are necessary to provide optimum care. Successful resuscitation, however, requires not only that those involved in the attempt apply their knowledge and skills quickly and appropriately. This chapter deals both with the correct application of knowledge and skills and with the control of the resuscitation attempt.

THE SEQUENCE OF MANAGEMENT OF CARDIOPULMONARY RESUSCITATION

The ideal sequence for cardiac resuscitation is shown in Figure 11.1. This sequence is designed to optimize the outcome by ensuring that both diagnosis and basic life support precede advanced cardiac life support, and also that advanced techniques and treatments are carried out in the most efficacious order. If more than one member of the resuscitation team is capable of performing advanced techniques, then some tasks may be carried out concurrently; however, the overall order should still be followed.

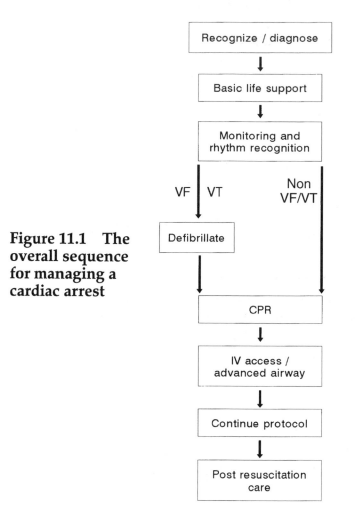

Figure 11.1 The overall sequence for managing a cardiac arrest

Recognition and diagnosis

It is essential that a cardiopulmonary collapse is recognized swiftly and diagnosed accurately, since these two steps must precede the administration of basic life support. Many people (even professional healthcare providers) have surprising difficulty in persuading themselves that a patient has suffered cardiopulmonary collapse; this is presumably because of the embarrassment they would feel if wrong. Since time to basic life support is so critical in determining outcome, every effort must be made to fight against this tendency 'to be absolutely sure'. By applying the methods of assessment discussed in Chapter 5 (the SAFE approach, evaluate ABC) these delays can be avoided. It is always better to overdiagnose and be embarrassed than to underdiagnose and reduce the chances of a good outcome.

Basic life support

It is important that BLS is applied as quickly and effectively as possible, and that **it is continued throughout the resuscitation attempt**. Cardiac and respiratory support should never be discontinued for more than 10 s (except during defibrillation) from the time the diagnosis is made, until either spontaneous circulation and breathing return, or the attempt at resuscitation is formally abandoned. Failure to provide continuous good BLS greatly decreases the chance of a favourable outcome.

The techniques of BLS are discussed in detail in Chapter 5.

Monitoring

Since ventricular fibrillation is common and treatable, and time is important, an accurate diagnosis of the rhythm must be made as early as possible and the patient quickly attached to an ECG monitor. The use of paddle electrodes and the advent of automatic and advisory defibrillators have made the technique of 'blind defibrillation' (defibrillation carried out before monitoring of any sort) very rare.

Defibrillation and rhythm diagnosis

Defibrillation

If ventricular fibrillation is diagnosed, defibrillation is the single most efficacious treatment. Furthermore, as discussed in Chapter 1, the time to delivery of the first DC shock is critical in determining outcome. It follows, therefore, that defibrillation should be the first manoeuvre to be considered in the advanced cardiac life support of cardiac arrest.

In ventricular fibrillation and pulseless ventricular tachycardia a rapid sequence of three attempts at defibrillation should precede all other advanced interventions. Between shocks, the paddles should be left on the patient's chest while the defibrillator is recharged. The pulse in the carotid artery should be checked only if the rhythm on the monitor changes to one normally associated with a spontaneous circulation. BLS should be provided between shocks only if the time to charge the defibrillator is excessive. If the rhythm appears to be asystole but ventricular fibrillation cannot be excluded, the same sequence should be followed.

Defibrillation is discussed in detail in Chapter 16.

Rhythm diagnosis

If ventricular fibrillation and pulseless ventricular tachycardia can be excluded the rhythm should be diagnosed while airway control and/or vascular access are being achieved (see below).

Dysrhythmia recognition is discussed in detail in Chapter 8.

Endotracheal intubation and vascular access

If immediate defibrillation is not indicated or has failed and adequate basic life support is being performed, the next priority is to establish a route for drug administration. Adrenaline is the first drug given in all the cardiac arrest protocols, and can be given by the intravenous or tracheal route. Therefore either endotracheal intubation or central venous cannulation may be carried out. If the patient has not arrested, and does not therefore require intubation or a central venous line, peripheral intravenous access should be established.

The choice between intubation and venous access for giving adrenaline should be made by the team leader, taking into account both the condition of the patient and the skills of the team members. In general, if skills are limited and procedures cannot be carried out concurrently, tracheal intubation using a cuffed tube should be performed before central venous access because of the additional protection offered to the airway, and the initial dose of adrenaline is given via the trachea. External chest compression and ventilation should then be continued.

If more than one person is participating in the resuscitation, a central line may now be established (or the trachea intubated) without interruption of CPR. However, when only one person is carrying out the resuscitation, the remaining procedure should be attempted after delivery of the next three shocks.

If tracheal intubation or venous access is difficult, CPR must not be interrupted for more than 15 s, and adrenaline should continue to be given via the route available. Endotracheal intubation and central venous cannulation are described in Chapter 14 and Chapter 15, respectively.

Continuing the treatment protocol

The treatment protocol for the diagnosed rhythm should be followed. Adrenaline should be given every 3 min during the resuscitation attempt.

Treatment protocols are discussed in detail in Chapter 9.

Reassessment

Throughout resuscitation constant attention should be given to checking that basic life support is still adequate. The rhythm should be monitored for changes, and the functioning of equipment checked.

Post-resuscitation care

Even if adequate spontaneous circulation returns the airway and ventilation may still require support. Arterial blood gas analysis should be performed urgently. Pharmacological agents may be needed to try and prevent dysrhythmias recurring.

The immediate diagnostic work-up should be commenced as soon as possible, and referral made to the appropriate in-patient facility.

Blood gas interpretation is dealt with in Chapter 4, and post-resuscitation care is discussed in more detail in Chapter 10.

THE RESUSCITATION TEAM

Team size and the mix of skills within the team will vary widely according to circumstances. Some of the various tasks that may be allocated to team members are shown in Box 11.1.

Box 11.1   Tasks that may be allocated to team members

Airway control and ventilation

External cardiac massage

Defibrillation and rhythm recognition

Establishment of intravascular access

Drug administration

Management of drug and other supplies

Documentation

Liaison

Counselling of relatives

Some of these tasks can be carried out by staff without special skills, others require staff with appropriate training. If only one member of the team is trained in advanced techniques then strict adherence to the sequence of events outlined above is essential. If a more skilled team has been assembled then some of the tasks may be addressed concurrently by different team members.

THE TEAM LEADER

One member of the team must assume the role of team leader. If only one person is an advanced cardiac life support provider, the choice of leader is simple. If a team that has more skilled personnel is likely to be present, then the name of the team leader should be clearly stated before the team is on call.

The team leader should be in control of the situation, and should co-ordinate the actions of the team members. The responsibilities of the team leader are shown in Box 11.2.

Box 11.2   Responsibilities of the team leader

Directing the team

Checking that assigned tasks are carried out correctly

Ensuring the safety of team members

Assessing the patient

Solving problems

Making the final decision to abandon resuscitation

Direction

Only the team leader should give orders during the resuscitation. This does not exclude other team members from making suggestions, but implies that the final decision rests with the leader.

It is desirable for the team leader to 'stand back' in order to view and direct the whole resuscitation attempt, rather than becoming personally involved in solving individual problems. This is easier if there are a number of skilled people in the team, and very difficult if the leader is also the only skilled person. In the latter case the leader should make deliberate attempts to review the whole resuscitation at regular intervals, in order to check that nothing vital is being missed.

Supervision

The supervision of the team involves ensuring that both basic life support and advanced cardiac life support are being provided correctly, and according to the orders given. Specific points that should be watched for are shown in Box 11.3.

Box 11.3   Points the team leader should watch for

Adequacy of external cardiac compression

Correct ratio in basic life support

Maintenance of adequate basic life support

Correct and safe defibrillation technique

Assessment of pulse following defibrillation

Correct choice and use of airway adjuncts

Correct ventilator settings

Correct choice and placement of intravascular access

Correct monitor control settings

Correct drugs administered

In general, then, the team leader must be everywhere and check everything.

Safety

The leader also has the responsibility for ensuring that team members are safe. This is particularly important in the out-of-hospital environment, and when potentially hazardous procedures such as defibrillation are being performed.

Patient assessment

Since assessment of the patient is the key to correct decision making, this task is also the responsibility of the team leader. First, the history of the arrest should be established. This can be obtained from nursing and paramedical staff. Pertinent facts include:

● Where

● When

● Witnessed or not

● Time to basic life support

● Initial rhythm

● Time to defibrillation

● Special circumstances

● Other therapeutic interventions

The past medical history and drug history should be sought. This is more easily obtained for in-patients. In out-of-hospital arrest relatives may be present or, if not, an urgent retrieval of old hospital notes and a call to the general practitioner can provide invaluable information. Patients often carry prescription cards with them, although the accuracy of these is sometimes doubtful.

The team leader should also discover whether current signed and dated 'not for resuscitation' orders are in force.

Solving problems

If the patient fails to respond to interventions as expected, then it is the team leader's responsibility to investigate, decide why, and initiate appropriate changes to treatment. This may involve, amongst other things, reassessing the original diagnosis, recognizing equipment malfunction or recognizing misplacement of lines or tubes.

The team leader is also responsible for the interpretation of the results of investigations, and initiation of therapy based on them as appropriate.

Deciding to stop

The decision to stop is always difficult. However, once the diagnosis has been confirmed, the correct treatment protocols applied, compounding problems such as hypothermia treated, and all relevant history gathered, the team leader should be in a position to decide. It is the team leader's responsibility to make the final decision, but it is usual to discuss this with the rest of the team before stopping.

SUMMARY

The ideal sequence for adult resuscitation should be followed. Some aspects may be performed concurrently if sufficient skilled personnel are present. The resuscitation team has a large number of tasks to perform – to perform them optimally the resuscitation should be controlled by a team leader.

SECTION THREE
Special situations

────12────
Paediatric life support

Objectives

After reading this chapter you should be able to:

- Understand the pathophysiology of cardiac arrest in childhood

- Understand the principles of paediatric basic life support

- Understand the principles of paediatric advanced cardiac life support

CAUSES OF CARDIAC ARREST IN CHILDHOOD

Most deaths in infancy and childhood occur in previously well children. In the newborn period the most common causes of death are due either to factors associated with prematurity (e.g. respiratory immaturity, cerebral haemorrhage, or infection due to immaturity of the immune response), or to congenital abnormalities.

In the first year of life the condition described as 'cot death' is the most common cause of death. Some infant victims of this condition have previously unrecognized respiratory or metabolic diseases, while in others no adequate explanation for death is found at detailed post-mortem examination. This latter group of children are described as victims of the sudden infant death syndrome (SIDS). After the age of one, trauma is the most common cause of death and remains so until well into early adult life.

Cardiac arrest in infancy and childhood is rarely due to primary cardiac disease. The majority of cases are secondary to hypoxia. This may have resulted from conditions such as birth asphyxia, epiglottitis, inhalation of foreign body, bronchiolitis, asthma or pneumothorax. Whatever the cause, by the time cardiac arrest occurs the child has had a period of respiratory insufficiency which will have caused respiratory acidosis (from carbon dioxide retention), and metabolic acidosis (from hypoxia) (see Chapter 4). This combination of hypoxia and acidosis will have caused cell damage and death in sensitive organs such as the brain, liver and kidney, well before myocardial damage is severe enough to cause cardiac arrest.

The other major underlying cause of cardiac arrest is circulatory failure (shock). This will have resulted from either blood loss or fluid redistribution. The former is due to trauma, the latter may be the result of conditions such as gastroenteritis, burns, sepsis, or anaphylaxis. The end point once again is tissue hypoxia, metabolic acidosis and cardiac arrest. The pathways leading to cardiac arrest in children are summarized in Figure 12.1.

**Figure 12.1
Pathways
leading to
cardiac arrest in
childhood**

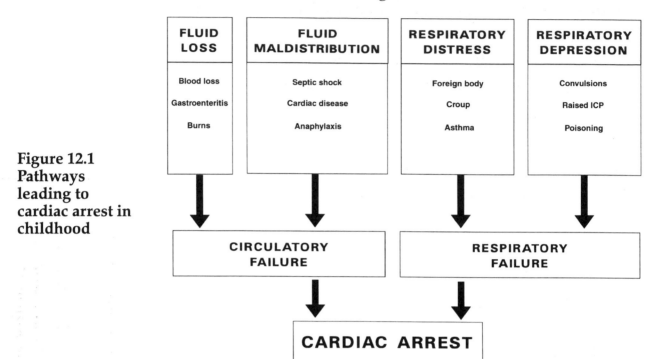

The aetiology of cardiac arrest in children should be contrasted with that in adults, where the primary cause of arrest is usually cardiac. Cardiorespiratory function may be near normal until the time that the arrest occurs. Consequently, in adults, hypoxia and ischaemic tissue damage occur **after** the heart has stopped and may therefore be prevented by prompt treatment.

The worst outcome is in children who arrive apnoeic and pulseless at the emergency department. These patients have a less than 5% chance of intact neurological survival, since there has often been a prolonged period of hypoxia and ischaemia prior to cardiopulmonary resuscitation. Earlier recognition and treatment of seriously ill children, and more widespread paediatric CPR training, could improve the outcome.

RECOGNITION OF RESPIRATORY AND CIRCULATORY FAILURE

As the outcome from cardiac arrest in childhood is so poor, it is vital to recognize the signs of respiratory and/or circulatory failure whatever their cause before the arrest occurs.

The following signs are suggestive of respiratory failure:

- Tachypnoea
- Use of accessory muscles of respiration
- Severe chest retraction
- Decreased or absent breath sounds
- Restlessness and agitation or decreased level of consciousness
- Hypotonia
- Cyanosis (this is a late and preterminal sign)

The following signs are suggestive of circulatory failure:

- Rapid thready pulse
- Rapid deep breathing
- Agitation or depressed conscious level
- Skin pallor and coldness with poor capillary refill
- Oliguria
- Hypotension (late sign)

BASIC LIFE SUPPORT IN CHILDREN

Introduction

Paediatric basic life support is not simply a scaled-down version of that provided for adults. Although the general principles are the same, specific techniques are required if the optimum support is to be given. Furthermore the exact techniques employed need to be varied according to the size of the child. A somewhat artificial line is generally drawn between infants (less than 1 year old) and small children (less than 8 years old), and that approach is followed here.

By applying the basic techniques described, a single rescuer can support the vital respiratory and circulatory functions of a collapsed child with no equipment.

The SAFE approach

On discovering or being asked to help to care for a collapsed child, **Shout** to summon help. The arrival of assistance will help with performing BLS and allow earlier summoning of advanced help via the telephone. It is essential that the rescuer does not become a second victim, and the rescuer must **Approach** with care and ensure that the child is **Free** from any continuing danger. These considerations should precede the initial **Evaluation** of the patient's Airway, Breathing and Circulation.

159

Summary

When dealing with a collapsed child:

Shout for help

Approach with care

Free from danger

Evaluate ABC

PATIENT EVALUATION

Are you all right?

As in adults, the initial simple assessment of responsiveness consists of asking the child 'Are you all right?', and gently shaking them by the shoulders. Infants and very small children who cannot yet talk, and older children who are very scared, are unlikely to reply meaningfully although they may make some sound or open their eyes to the rescuer's voice.

In cases associated with trauma the neck and spine should be immobilized during this manoeuvre. This is achieved by placing one hand firmly on the forehead, while gently shaking one of the child's arms.

Assessment and treatment

Once the child has been approached correctly and a simple test for unresponsiveness has been carried out, assessment and treatment follow the ABC pattern. The overall sequence of basic life support in cardio-pulmonary arrest is summarized in Figure 12.2.

Airway

An obstructed airway may be the primary problem, and correction of the obstruction can result in recovery without further intervention.

If a child is having difficulty breathing, but is conscious, then transport to hospital should be arranged as quickly as possible. A child will often find the best position to maintain their own airway, and should not be forced to adopt a position which they find less comfortable. Attempts to improve a partially maintained airway in an environment where immediate advanced support is not available can be dangerous, since total obstruction may occur.

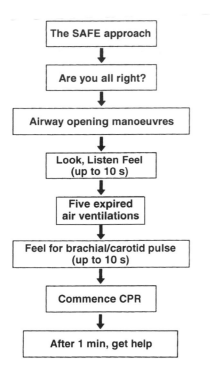

Figure 12.2 The sequence of basic life support in children

If the child is unconscious then steps must be taken to ensure that their airway is open.

The airway is most commonly blocked by the tongue falling back to obstruct the pharynx. An attempt to open the airway should be made using head tilt/chin lift. The rescuer places the hand nearest to the child's head on the forehead, and applies pressure to gently tilt the head back. The desirable degrees of tilt are:

Infant Neutral

Child Sniffing

The fingers of the other hand should then be placed under the chin, which is then lifted upwards. Care should be taken not to injure the soft tissue of the floor of the mouth by gripping too hard. Since this action can close the child's mouth, it may be necessary to use the thumb of the same hand to part the lips slightly. The optimal position for airway opening in infants is shown in Figure 12.3.

An alternative to the head tilt/chin lift is the jaw thrust. This is achieved by placing two or three fingers under the angle of the mandible bilaterally, and lifting the jaw upwards. The technique may be easier if the rescuer's elbows are resting on the same surface as the child is lying on. A small degree of head tilt may also be applied.

It should be noted that if there is a history of trauma then the head tilt/chin lift manoeuvre may exacerbate cervical spine injury. The safest airway intervention in these circumstances is jaw thrust without head tilt. Proper cervical spine control can be achieved in

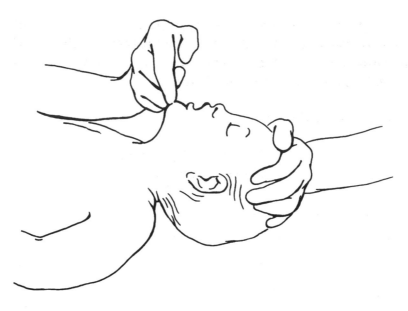

**Figure 12.3
Airway opening
in infants**

such cases only by a second rescuer maintaining in-line cervical stabilization throughout.

The finger sweep technique often recommended in adults should not be used in children. The child's soft palate is easily damaged and bleeding from within the mouth can worsen the situation. Furthermore foreign bodies may be forced further down the airway; these can get lodged below the cords and become even more difficult to remove.

If a foreign body is not obvious, inspection of the upper airway should be carried out under direct vision in hospital, and if appropriate, removal should be attempted using Magill forceps.

Breathing

Once these manoeuvres have been carried out the presence or absence of breathing should be assessed. This is achieved by the rescuer placing his face above the child's, with his ear over the nose, the cheek over the mouth, and his eyes looking along the line of the child's chest:

- LOOKing for chest movement.
- LISTENing for breath sounds.
- FEELing for expired air.

If the airway opening techniques described above do not result in the resumption of breathing, exhaled air resuscitation should be commenced.

While the airway is kept open as described above, the rescuer breathes in and seals his mouth around the child's mouth, or mouth and nose. If the mouth alone is used then the nose should be pinched closed using the thumb and index fingers of the hand that is maintaining head tilt. Slow exhalation (1–1.5 s) by the rescuer should result in the victim's chest rising.

Five initial rescue breaths should be given

Since children vary in size only general guidance can be given regarding the volume and pressure of inflation.

- The chest should be seen to rise.
- Inflation pressure may be higher since airways are small.
- Slow breaths at the lowest pressure reduce gastric distension.

If the chest does not rise then the airway is not clear. The usual cause is failure to carry out the airway opening techniques correctly. Therefore the first thing to do is to readjust the head tilt/chin lift position, and try again. If this does not work jaw thrust should be tried. If two rescuers are present one should maintain the airway while the other breathes for the child. Failure of both head tilt/chin lift and jaw thrust should lead to the suspicion that a foreign body is causing the obstruction, and appropriate action should be taken. This is discussed later.

An assessment of the circulation must now be made.

Circulation

Feel for the presence and rate of the pulse for up to 10 s. In infants the neck is generally short and fat, and the carotid artery may be difficult to identify. Therefore the brachial artery should be felt in the medial aspect of the antecubital fossa (Figure 12.4). In small children, as in adults, the carotid artery can be palpated in the neck.

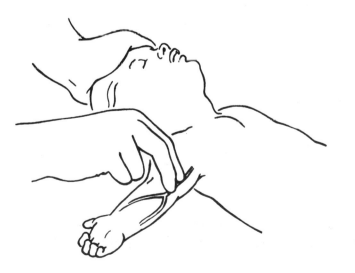

**Figure 12.4
Feeling for the
brachial pulse**

163

If the pulse is present and at an adequate rate (over 60 beats/min) but apnoea persists, exhaled air resuscitation must be continued until spontaneous breathing resumes. If the pulse is inadequate in infants or young children (less than 60 beats/min) or absent in older children, external cardiac compression is required.

Cardiac compression

For the best output the child must be placed lying flat on their back, on a hard surface. In infants it is said that the palm of the rescuer's hand can be used for this purpose, but this may prove difficult in practice.

Children vary in size, and the exact nature of the compressions given should reflect this. In general, infants (less than 1 year) require a different technique from small children. In children over 8 years of age the method used in adults can be applied with appropriate modifications for their size.

Infants

Since the infant heart is lower in relation to external landmarks than in older children and adults, the area of compression is found by imagining a line between the nipples and compressing over the sternum one finger's breadth below this line. Two fingers are used to compress the chest to a depth of approximately 1.5–2.5 cm. This is shown in Figure 12.5.

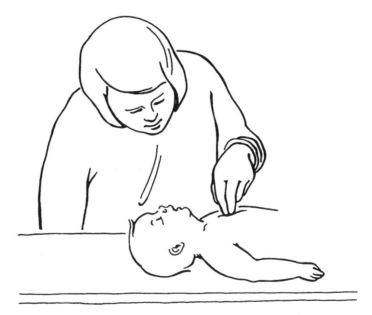

**Figure 12.5
Chest
compressions in
an infant**

Alternatively, infant cardiac compression can be achieved using the hand encircling technique. The infant is held with both the rescuer's hands encircling the chest. The thumbs are placed over the correct part of the sternum (see above) and compression carried out.

Small children

The area of compression is one finger's breadth above the xiphisternum. The heel of one hand is used to compress the sternum to a depth of approximately 2.5–3.5 cm (see Figure 12.6).

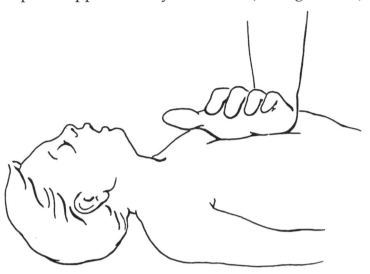

Figure 12.6 Chest compressions in small children

Larger children

The area of compression is two fingers' breadths above the xiphisternum. The heels of both hands are used to compress the sternum to a depth of approximately 3–4.5 cm, depending on the size of the child. This is illustrated in Figure 12.7.

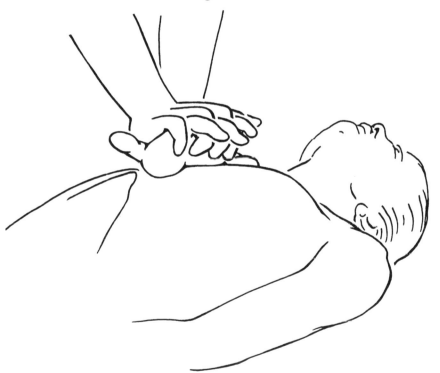

Figure 12. 7 Chest compressions in older children

Once the correct technique has been chosen and the area for compression identified

Five external chest compressions should be given

Cardiopulmonary resuscitation is now continued using a ratio of one expired air ventilation to five chest compressions, irrespective of the number of rescuers. Since the normal heart rate in infants and children is higher than in adults, the optimal compression rate is higher – 100/min. The aim should be to achieve 20 cycles (1:5) per minute.

Basic life support must not be interrupted

Any time spent in readjusting the airway or reestablishing the correct position for compressions will seriously decrease the number of cycles given per minute. This can be a very real problem for the solo rescuer and there is no easy solution. However, slower rates performed efficiently are preferred.

If in an older child effective chest compression can be achieved only by using a two-handed technique, then a single rescuer should use a ratio of 2 breaths to 15 compressions, aiming for a rate of 80–100 compressions per minute.

The single rescuer should continue basic life support for 1 min before summoning help. Although this may mean leaving an older child, infants and small children may be carried to the telephone, minimizing interruption of BLS.

The CPR manoeuvres recommended for infants and children are summarized in Table 12.1.

Table 12.1 Summary of BLS techniques in infants and children

	Age		
	Infants **<1 year**	**Small children** **1 – 8 years**	**Larger children** **>8 years**
Airway			
Head tilt position	Neutral	Sniffing	Sniffing
Breathing			
Initial slow breaths	5	5	5
Circulation			
Pulse check	Brachial	Carotid	Carotid
Landmark	One finger's breadth below nipple line	One finger's breadth above xiphisternum	Two fingers' breadths above xiphisternum
Technique	Two fingers or encircling	One hand	Two hands
Depth	1.5–2.5 cm	2.5–3.5 cm	3–4.5 cm
CPR			
Ratio	1:5	1:5	1:5 (2:15)
Cycles/min	20	20	20 (6)

The choking child

Introduction

The vast majority of deaths from foreign body aspiration occur in pre-school children. Virtually anything may be inhaled. The diagnosis is very rarely clear cut, but should be suspected if the onset of respiratory compromise is sudden and is associated with coughing, gagging and stridor. Airway obstruction may also occur with infections such as acute epiglottitis and croup. In such cases attempts to relieve the obstruction using the methods described below are dangerous. Children with known or suspected infectious causes of obstruction, and those who are still breathing and in whom the cause of obstruction is unclear, should be taken to hospital urgently. As discussed above, failure to establish an open airway despite simple manoeuvres should be taken to imply airway obstruction.

The physical methods of clearing the airway that are described below should be performed if:

- The diagnosis of foreign body aspiration is clear cut, and dyspnoea is increasing or apnoea has occurred.

- Head tilt/chin lift and jaw thrust have failed to open the airway of an apnoeic child.

Infants

There is concern that abdominal thrusts may cause intra-abdominal injury in infants. Therefore a combination of back blows and chest thrusts are recommended for the relief of foreign body obstruction in this age group.

The infant is placed along one of the rescuer's arms in a head down position. The rescuer then rests their arm along their thigh, and delivers five back blows with the heel of their free hand (Figure 12.8).

If the obstruction is not relieved the baby is turned over and laid supine along the rescuer's thigh, still in a head-down position. Five chest thrusts are given, using the same landmarks as for cardiac compression but a slower rate. The mouth should then be examined for any foreign body, the breathing assessed and, if inadequate or absent, expired air ventilation attempted before repeating the above cycle.

If an infant is too large to allow the single arm technique to be used, then the same manoeuvres can be performed by lying the baby across the rescuer's lap.

**Figure 12.8
Back blows in an
infant**

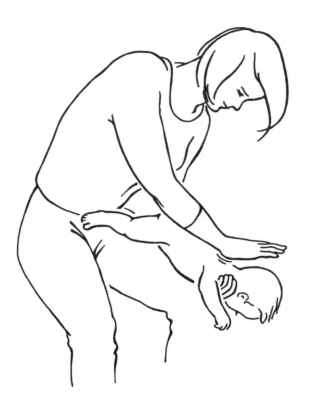

Children

In the older child, if five backblows fail the Heimlich manoeuvre may be used. As in the adult, this can be performed with the patient standing, sitting, kneeling or lying.

The rescuer moves behind the child and passes their arms around them. It may be necessary for an adult to stand the child on a box or other convenient object to carry out the standing manoeuvre effectively. One hand is formed into a fist and placed against the child's abdomen above the umbilicus and below the xiphisternum. The other hand is placed over the fist, and both hands are thrust sharply upwards into the abdomen. This is repeated five times unless the object causing the obstruction is expelled before then.

To carry out the Heimlich manoeuvre in a supine child, the rescuer kneels at their feet. If the child is large it may be necessary to kneel astride them. The heel of one hand is placed against the child's abdomen above the umbilicus and below the xiphisternum. The other hand is placed above the first, and both hands are thrust sharply downwards and upwards into the abdomen with care being taken to direct the thrust in the midline. This is repeated five times unless the object causing the obstruction is expelled before then. The mouth should then be examined for any foreign body, the breathing assessed and, if inadequate or absent, expired air ventilation attempted before repeating the above cycle.

Putting it all together: managing a choking child

The sequence of actions necessary to manage a choking child is shown in Figure 12.9.

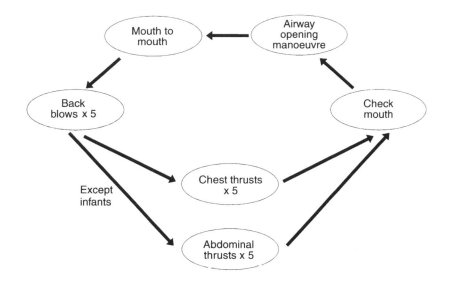

**Figure 12.9
Algorithm for
managing a
choking child**

ADVANCED SUPPORT OF THE AIRWAY AND VENTILATION

Airway and breathing assessment and resuscitation come first in the management of patients of all ages. If BLS techniques fail, it is vital that advanced techniques for obtaining a patent airway and achieving adequate ventilation and oxygenation are applied quickly and effectively.

Airway adjuncts

An oropharyngeal (Guedel) airway may be used to try to improve or provide a patent airway in the obtunded child. The oropharyngeal airway comes in a variety of sizes, from 000 for neonates to 1 for children (sizes 2–4 for adults). An estimate of the correct size can be made by comparing the airway with the vertical distance from the angle of the child's mouth to the ear lobe. Too small an airway will press against the tongue, while one that is too large will cause trauma.

In the older child the airway can be inserted 'upside down' as in adults. However, in babies and young children there is a danger that the soft palate may be damaged using this technique, and it is better to insert the airway the correct way up, under direct vision and using a tongue depressor or a laryngoscope to move the tongue. Despite taking care, an oropharyngeal airway may occasionally cause trauma and bleeding or laryngospasm and vomiting

169

if the gag reflex is present. After inserting an airway the patient should be assessed using look, listen and feel.

Nasopharyngeal airways are not widely used in children. This is partly because small sizes suitable for children are not made and therefore a tracheal tube of appropriate diameter has to be cut to length. Furthermore the vascular nasal mucosa and large adenoids are easily damaged during insertion and may bleed profusely.

Tracheal intubation

In the unresponsive child, the best method of securing the airway is by tracheal intubation. This will facilitate ventilation and protect against the risk of aspiration of regurgitated gastric contents or blood. The oral rather than the nasal route is preferred, for the reasons stated above. The practical procedure is described in Chapter 14.

Ventilation

Advanced ventilation consists of using either a self-inflating bag or a mechanical ventilator to deliver a high inspired oxygen concentration to the patient, 100% is the ideal.

Self-inflating bags are the most common devices used to ventilate apnoeic patients. Smaller volume bags of 240 ml and 500 ml are used for infants and children, respectively. They are fitted with a one-way valve to prevent rebreathing; and have a pressure limit (45 cmH$_2$O) to prevent the lungs suffering from barotrauma due to over-enthusiastic ventilation.

These bags can be connected either to a face mask of the appropriate size or to the tracheal tube directly via a catheter mount. When used on their own the patient is ventilated with air (21% oxygen), but the concentration can be raised to 50% by connecting an oxygen supply to an inlet adjacent to the air intake, and to 95% by using a reservoir bag or tubing.

It is important to remember that if a child-sized bag is not immediately available, an adult bag can be used if suitable adjustment is made in the tidal volume of gas delivered. The rates at which children should be ventilated are shown in Table 12.2.

Table 12.2 Ventilation rates

Age	Ventilatory rate/min
Neonates (less than 1 month)	60
Infant (less than 1 year)	30–40
1–8 years	20–30
>8 years	16
Adult	12

Mechanical ventilators can also be used to ventilate children of all ages. However, they are very powerful and if set incorrectly can deliver very large volumes of gas. This in turn can impair cardiac function and may cause severe pulmonary barotrauma. Consequently use of these devices is best left to the experts.

Whichever method of advanced ventilation is used, it is important to check that the lungs are being adequately ventilated by looking for chest movement and listening for breath sounds.

The surgical airway

Needle cricothyroidotomy

Cricothyroidotomy is a 'technique of failure', and as such should be used only when all other means of obtaining an airway have failed. This situation usually occurs following laryngeal obstruction from a foreign body, inflammation or tumour, or following major trauma. Although cricothyroidotomy is rarely needed, it can be life-saving, and must be performed promptly when indicated. The technique is simple in concept but far from easy in practice, and not without hazard.

Needle cricothyroidotomy is preferred to surgical cricothyroidotomy in children under 12 years old, since damage to the cricoid cartilage (which is the only complete ring of cartilage supporting the trachea) is usually avoided. The techniques are described in Chapter 14.

Transtracheal insufflation is a temporizing measure since, although oxygenation can be achieved, carbon dioxide will accumulate and render the child acidotic. Urgent arrangements must be made to perform a definitive tracheostomy.

THE MANAGEMENT OF CARDIAC ARREST

Cardiac arrest has occurred when there are no palpable central pulses. Basic life support with optimal oxygenation (preferably by intubation and ventilation) and with chest compressions must be established immediately. It must not be interrupted for more than 10 s until satisfactory cardiac output has been restored, except to defibrillate.

The following arrest rhythms are discussed in this section:

- Asystole

- Ventricular fibrillation

- Electromechanical dissociation

Drugs need to be given according to the weight of the child. This can be calculated (for children from 1 to 10 years of age) using the formula

2(age + 4)

Alternatively a height-to-weight nomogram (such as in the Broselow tape) or an age-to-weight nomogram (as in the Oakley chart) can be used.

Asystole

This is the most common arrest rhythm in children. The response of the young heart to prolonged severe hypoxia and acidosis is progressive bradycardia leading to asystole (Figure 12.10).

Figure 12.10 Asystole

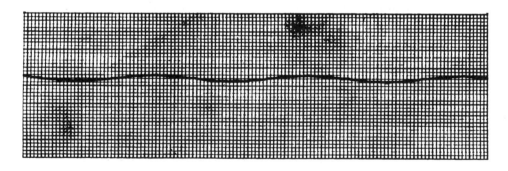

The algorithm for management of asystole in a child is shown in Figure 12.11.

Adrenaline is the first-line drug for asystole. The initial intravenous dose is 10 μg/kg (0.1 ml/kg of a 1:10 000 solution). This is best given through a central line, but if one is not in place it may be given through a peripheral or intraosseous line followed by a normal saline flush (2–5 ml). If there is no vascular access, the endotracheal

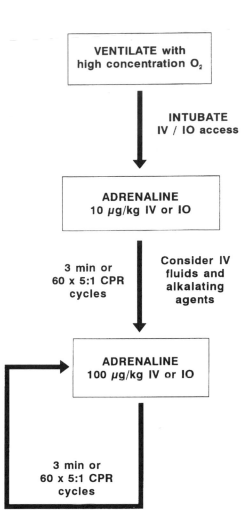

Figure 12.11 Algorithm for management of asystole in children

tube can be used at ten times the intravenous dose (i.e. 100 μg/kg). The drug should be injected quickly down a narrow-bore suction catheter beyond the tracheal end of the tube and then flushed in with 1 or 2 ml normal (0.9%) saline. In patients with pulmonary disease or prolonged asystole, pulmonary oedema and intrapulmonary shunting may make the endotracheal route less effective and 0.1 ml/kg of a 1:1000 solution should be used. If there has been no clinical effect, further doses should be given intravenously as soon as venous access has been secured.

Children with asystole may be profoundly acidotic as their cardiac arrest has usually been preceded by respiratory arrest or shock. The routine use of alkalizing agents has not been shown to be of benefit and should be administered only if profound acidosis is likely, and after the first dose of adrenaline has not caused the return of spontaneous circulation. In the arrested patient arterial pH does not correlate well with tissue pH (see Chapter 4). Therefore mixed venous or central venous pH should be used to guide any alkalizing therapy. It must also be remembered that good basic life support is more effective than alkalizing agents at correcting the acidosis. Bicarbonate is the most common alkalizing agent currently available, the dose being 1 mmol/kg (1 ml/kg of an 8.4% solution). The tracheal route should be avoided, and interactions with other drugs must be borne in mind.

In some situations, where the cardiac arrest has resulted from circulatory failure, a standard (20 ml/kg) bolus of fluid should be given if there is no response to the initial dose of adrenaline. The nature of the fluid is less important than the volume, and either a crystalloid such as normal (physiological) saline, or a colloid such as 5% human albumin can be given.

A second bolus of adrenaline (at a dose of ten times the first – 0.1 ml/kg of 1:1000) should be given if spontaneous cardiac output has not returned. If there is still no response, high-dose adrenaline should be administered every 3 min (60 × 1:5 CPR cycles). A continuous infusion of adrenaline at 2 μg/kg/min may be tried as an alternative to this. Evidence suggests that the outcome of asystole in childhood is very poor if there is no response to the second dose of adrenaline. There is no evidence that calcium is helpful, in fact calcium can be detrimental, causing coronary artery spasm. Consequently it must be used only to treat documented hypocalcaemia, hyperkalaemia or hypermagnesaemia.

Ventricular fibrillation

Figure 12.12 Ventricular fibrillation

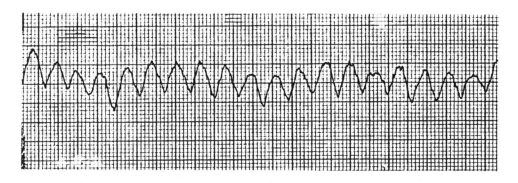

This rhythm is uncommon in children but should be sought in those who are recovering from hypothermia, those poisoned by tricyclic antidepressants and those with cardiac disease. The algorithm for management of ventricular fibrillation (VF) in a child is shown in Figure 12.13.

Electrical defibrillation must be carried out immediately. Paediatric paddles (4.5 cm diameter or equivalent area) should be used for children under 10 kg. One electrode is placed just below the right clavicle and the other in the left mid-clavicular line at the level of the xiphoid. If only adult paddles are available for an infant under 10 kg, one may be placed on the infant's back and one over the left lower part of the chest at the front.

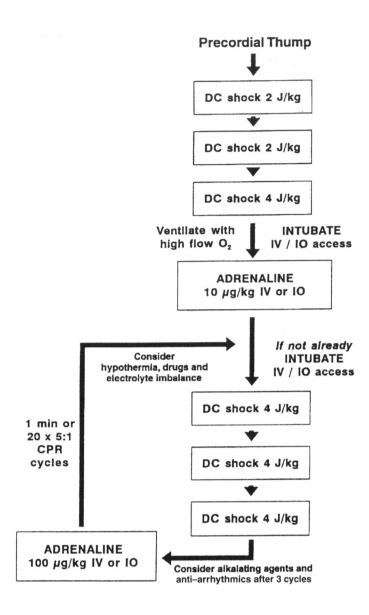

**Figure 12.13
Algorithm for
management of
VF in children**

The first two shocks should be at 2 J/kg, and the third at 4 J/kg. If these three shocks fail to produce defibrillation the patient should be hyperventilated (to increase pH), given adrenaline 10 μg/kg intravenously, and the shock (4 J/kg) repeated three times. This cycle is repeated with an adrenaline dose of 100 μg/kg. Different paddle positions or another defibrillator may be tried. Finally after nine shocks the anti-arrhythmic agents lignocaine, amiodarone or bretylium tosylate (5 mg/kg) may be used with further defibrillation attempts. Basic life support must be maintained throughout.

Electromechanical dissociation (EMD)

This is defined as absence of a palpable pulse, with recognizable complexes seen on the ECG monitor. The most common cause in children is profound shock which makes the pulse difficult to feel. The algorithm for treatment of electromechanical dissociation in children is shown in Figure 12.14.

175

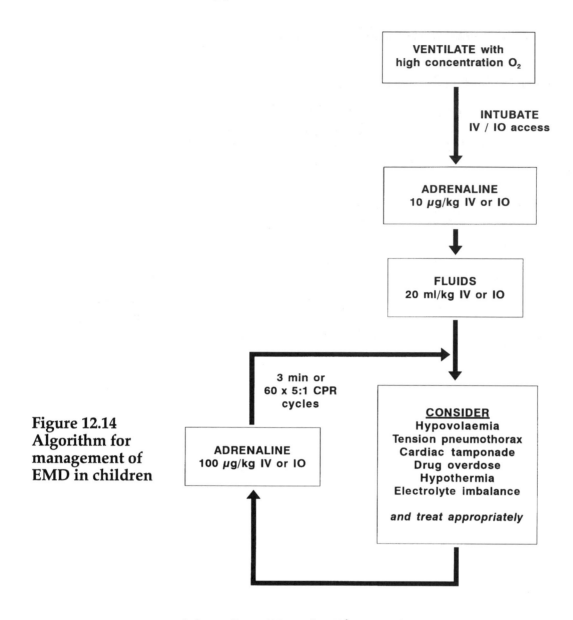

Figure 12.14 Algorithm for management of EMD in children

Adrenaline (10 μg/kg IV) must be given immediately. Rapid volume expansion with 20 ml/kg of crystalloid should then be commenced.

In patients who have suffered trauma, both cardiac tamponade and tension pneumothorax should be considered as causes of EMD and treated as discussed in Chapter 9.

Very occasionally, intravenous calcium may be required in a patient with EMD due to hypocalcaemia, hyperkalaemia, hypermagnesaemia or calcium channel blocker overdose. In this event patients should be treated with intravenous calcium chloride 10%, 10 mg/kg (0.1 ml/kg). The drug should be given slowly into a peripheral vein. Continuous monitoring is essential because calcium can give rise to bradycardia, coronary artery spasm and myocardial irritability. It can also cause severe local tissue damage if not given intravenously.

Adrenaline 100 μg/mg IV should be repeated every 60 CPR cycles.

OTHER DYSRHYTHMIAS IN CHILDHOOD

Supraventricular tachycardia (SVT)

This gives rise to a heart rate over 200 beats/min, and often up to 300 beats/min. The rhythm is regular and the QRS complexes are uniform in appearance. Each QRS is preceded by a P wave but this may not be apparent due to the tachycardia (Figure 12.15).

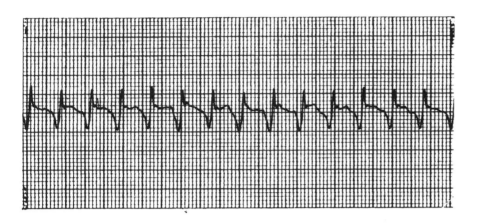

Figure 12.15 Supraventricular tachycardia

The onset and cessation are sudden. The rhythm may last for minutes or up to several days. It is tolerated remarkably well by some children, but an infant may present with sweating, poor colour, peripheral vasoconstriction, hepatomegaly and other signs of cardiac failure.

Unstable SVT

If the child is clinically shocked synchronized DC cardioversion must be used. The first shock should be given at 0.5–1.0 J/kg, with further ones being at 2.0 J/kg.

Ventricular tachycardia

This is defined as three or more ectopic ventricular beats, and is sustained if it continues for longer than 30 s. The rate varies between 120 and 250 beats/min (Figure 12.16).

It is not a common presenting rhythm in children without an underlying congenital heart disorder, myocarditis, or cardiomyopathy. The onset may be sudden, with rapid deterioration in tissue perfusion. This rhythm may degenerate into VF.

Unstable ventricular tachycardia

The unstable child should be given an unsynchronized DC shock.

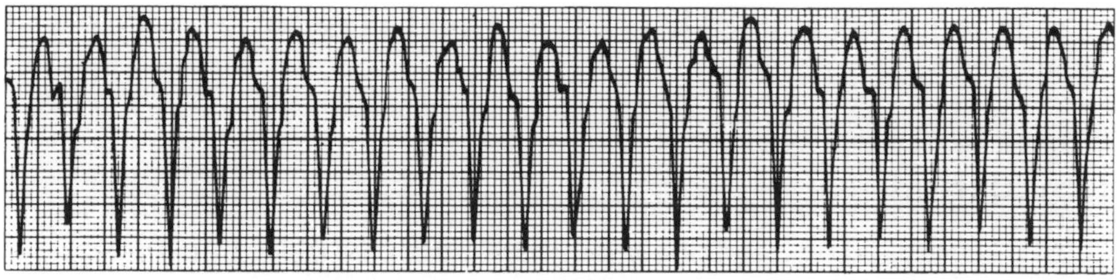

**Figure 12.16
Ventricular
tachycardia**

The first shock should be at 0.5–1.0 J/kg and should be followed by a bolus of IV lignocaine. Further shocks may be required, and should be given at 2.0 J/kg. An infusion of lignocaine may also be necessary.

Bradycardia in an unstable child

Hypoxia and shock must be treated first. Should the arrhythmia persist atropine 20 μg/kg (minimum 100 μg), can be given after this and the use of adrenaline (10 μg/kg) and pacing should be considered.

POST-RESUSCITATION CARE

Once ventilation and spontaneous cardiac output have been established, it is essential that frequent clinical reassessment is carried out. Ventilatory and circulatory adequacy, and consciousness level must be monitored to detect deterioration or improvement with therapy. All patients should be monitored as shown in Table 12.3.

Table 12.3: Methods of monitoring patients

Pulse rate and rhythm	ECG monitor
Oxygen saturation	Pulse oximeter
Core temperature	Low reading thermometer
Blood pressure	Non-invasive monitor
Urine output	Urinary catheter
Arterial pH and gases	Arterial blood sample

Additionally, some patients will require CO_2 monitoring, invasive BP monitoring, and central venous pressure monitoring

Airway and breathing

Most recently resuscitated children will have an impaired consciousness level and depressed gag reflex. They should remain intubated and ventilated to maintain oxygen saturation above 95% and keep blood gases as near normal as possible. Most survivors will be transferred to an ICU where ventilation can be adjusted as appropriate.

Circulation

Following cardiac arrest, cardiac output will usually be impaired by one or more of the following causes:

- Underlying cardiac abnormality
- Hypoxia, acidosis and toxins
- Acid–base or electrolyte disturbance
- Hypovolaemia

Arterial pH, oxygenation and electrolyte abnormalities should be identified and corrected. Hypoglycaemia should be sought and treated. Hypovolaemia should be treated by infusing 20 ml/kg of crystalloid or colloid. Following this, there may be a need for further circulatory expansion, inotropic drug support of the myocardium or vasodilatation of the circulatory system.

The placement of a central venous pressure line will assist in deciding whether to give more fluid, or inotropic support.

Cerebral management

Hypoxia and ischaemia occurring before cardiac arrest may have already caused brain damage. It is important to avoid further damage during the post-resuscitation period. This can be achieved by the following measures:

- Good oxygenation
- Normal blood pressure and perfusion
- Normal acid–base balance and electrolytes
- Normal blood sugar
- Normothermia
- Avoid unpleasant procedures without analgesia
- Normal intracranial pressure

Other considerations

Hypothermia

Sick or injured children become cold easily. Keep the child covered or under an infra red heater and monitor rectal temperature.

Hypoglycaemia

Sick infants have poor glycogen stores: glucose may need to be given during the course of CPR as indicated by stick tests. The dose is 0.5 g/kg IV.

WHEN TO STOP RESUSCITATION

If there have been no detectable signs of cardiac output and no evidence of cerebral activity despite 30 min CPR, it is reasonable to stop resuscitation. The decision will be taken by the team leader.

The exception is the hypothermic patient, in whom resuscitation must continue until the core temperature has reached at least 32°C, or in whom no detectable rise in core temperature can be achieved despite internal rewarming.

SUMMARY

Paediatric resuscitation from cardiac arrest reflects the different underlying primary events leading to the arrest. Correction of hypoxia is a key to successful resuscitation, while the need for defibrillation is low. The principles of basic and advanced life support are otherwise similar to those applied to the resuscitation of adults.

———13———
Special situations

Objectives

After reading this chapter you should be able to:

- Understand the variations in basic life support necessary in some special situations
- Understand the variations in advanced cardiac life support necessary in some special situations
- Understand the variations in post-resuscitation care necessary in some special situations

---

The vast majority of patients who suffer a cardiorespiratory arrest can be treated successfully by proper application of the standard protocols. However, certain special situations require that modifications are made to some aspects of their care. This part of the book deals with some of these situations. These are:

1. Near drowning
2. Hypothermia
3. Pregnancy
4. Drug overdoses
5. Trauma
6. Electrical injury
7. Smoke inhalation
8. Volatile substance abuse
9. Anaphylaxis

Each is covered in the same way. First, some background information is given. Secondly, under the heading 'Special considerations', the reasons for the particular problems of the situation are stated. In this section and in the following two sections ('Basic life support' and 'Advanced life support') these problems are dealt with in the familiar 'ABC' manner. Finally any changes necessary in the post-resuscitation care phase are noted.

If a heading does not appear then management is not significantly different from the standard protocols.

NEAR DROWNING

Incidence

Near drowning is defined as an episode of suffocation by submersion followed by at least transient recovery. Its true incidence in the UK is unknown but there are 700 drowning episodes per year and, if the proportion of drowning to near drowning is the same as that in the USA, this suggests some 7700 cases. All ages are affected but it is most common in the second decade and in children under 4 years.

Aetiology and mechanism

Drowning in deep water may result from inability to swim or from exhaustion compounded by hypothermia. Trauma, especially to the cervical spine, may render even the strongest swimmers liable to drowning, as may air emboli in scuba divers. Medical conditions such as epilepsy, hypoglycaemia and intoxication with drugs or alcohol can cause drowning even in shallow water. Non-accidental submersion may occur especially in children.

During a drowning episode water enters the airway and breathing stops, but the heart continues to beat and maintain cerebral perfusion for some time. Eventually the circulatory system fails and the patient has a cardiac arrest. The continued cardiac output following the cessation of breathing, coupled with rapid hypothermia, may explain why some patients (especially children) can survive neurologically intact after long periods of submersion.

The main causes of late death in near-drowning episodes are respiratory failure and ischaemic brain damage.

Special considerations

The clinical picture seen in near drowning is not affected by whether submersion was in salt or fresh water.

General

A combined respiratory and metabolic acidosis is common immediately after near drowning. However, by the time the patient reaches the emergency department, spontaneous respiration may already have been started. If breathing is adequate at this stage only the metabolic acidosis will remain.

The electrolyte disturbance following the water absorption is usually minor and rarely clinically significant. Occasionally fresh water absorption can lead to anaemia due to haemolysis.

Renal failure can appear as a late consequence of hypoxia, hypotension, lactic acidosis and myoglobinuria.

> **Death cannot be declared until basic and advanced life support have been continued, without success, for 45 min and the core temperature is over 32°C. A longer time should be allowed for children**

Basic life support

Although life support can be rendered in water it is much more efficient (and safer for the rescuer) when administered on land.

SAFE

No untoward risks should be taken during the rescue, and all available aids (such as flotation devices) should be used.

ABC

A: There is a high incidence of neck injuries associated with drowning. Care must be taken to prevent exacerbation of any cervical injury by maintaining in-line stabilization of the neck. This should be continued even when the patient is being turned to clear away any vomitus. Airway opening manoeuvres should be restricted to jaw thrust, rather than head tilt, chin lift.

B: Mouth to nose or mouth resuscitation can be started immediately, but all effort should be made to get the patient quickly from the water. Draining water from the lungs makes little difference to the oxygen uptake but it does delay treatment and potentially jeopardizes an unstable neck.

Water enters some of the alveoli and washes out surfactant. Atelectasis results, along with ventilation–perfusion mismatch and damage to the alveolar–capillary membrane. Pulmonary oedema occurs in 75% of cases as a consequence of the surfactant loss, direct pulmonary injury, inflammatory contaminants in the water and cerebral hypoxia.

C: Hypothermia can occur, with consequent inability to feel central pulses even if they are present.

Advanced life support

ABC

A: In-line cervical stabilization is maintained while the airway is reassessed and secured as well as during intubation if this is required.

C: Usually volume support is not critical in these patients so any infusion should initially be slow. Hypothermia is usually accompanied by a bradycardia.

General

A low-reading thermometer should be used to assess core temperature. When appropriate, therapy for hypothermia should be commenced (see p. 185).

Post-resuscitation care

A full examination is required to rule out associated injuries including a pneumothorax and air emboli in divers. A nasogastric tube and urinary catheter should be inserted if the patient is not fully conscious. A chest radiograph is needed in all cases of near drowning because it does have a predictive value. Almost 50% of patients with an abnormal chest radiograph will require intubation and ventilation. The film may show perihilar infiltrates or pulmonary oedema. If pulmonary oedema develops positive pressure ventilation will be required. Fever is common in the first few hours, but systemic infection should be suspected if a pyrexia develops after 24 h. Once blood cultures have been taken intravenous antibiotics can then be started with the chosen agent being effective against Gram-negative organisms. Prophylactic antibiotics and steroids are not required but regular tracheal cultures and blood for cultures, electrolytes and white cell counts should be taken.

Patients who have nearly drowned can be divided into three groups.

1. Fully conscious, no respiratory distress and an insignificant history of immersion. Discharged home after 6 h if no abnormalities are found on examination of the chest, there is a normal chest radiograph and normal arterial blood gases (ABG) when the patient is breathing room air.
2. Conscious but mild/moderate respiratory distress. These patients require overnight observation in hospital. Provided there is no spinal injury, they should be managed on their side because they have a significant chance of vomiting.

3. Apnoeic, with a palpable pulse. These patients require admission to ICU with intubation, mechanical ventilation, haemodynamic monitoring and plasma expansion.

HYPOTHERMIA

Hypothermia has occurred when the core temperature falls below 35°C. It may complicate cardiac dysfunction arising from other causes, or may itself give rise to dysfunction. Hypothermia is divided into three grades according to the core temperature (Table 13.1).

Table 13.1 Grades of hypothermia, according to core temperature

Grade	Temperature (°C)
Mild	32–35
Moderate	30–32
Severe	<32

Aetiology and mechanism

Hypothermia can arise because of increased heat loss, decreased heat production, severe underlying disease, or from a combination of these mechanisms. Common causes underlying these are shown in Table 13.2.

Table 13.2 Causes of hypothermia

Increased heat loss	Decreased heat production	Underlying disease
Conduction:	Unconsciousness	Pancreatitis
Cold immersion	Hypothyroidism	
	Hypopituitarism	Bowel perforation
	Hypoglycaemia	
Convection:	Hypoadrenalism	Pneumonia
High winds	Old age	
Skin diseases	Children	
Burns	Hypothalamic lesion	
Vasodilatation:		Acute renal failure
Alcohol		
Drugs		
Infection		
Skin diseases		

The body has several protective mechanisms to prevent hypothermia developing should the environmental temperature fall. These involve reducing heat loss from the skin surface by vasoconstriction and behavioural responses (such as putting on more clothes). Heat production can also be enhanced by increasing metabolic rate and shivering.

If the environmental conditions overwhelm the normal protective system, or if these mechanisms fail, the core temperature will fall. The victim will then demonstrate signs and symptoms which are a combination of both the low temperature itself and the homeostatic mechanisms, as summarized in Table 13.3

Table 13.3   Signs of hypothermia by severity

Mild	Moderate	Severe
Pale cold skin	Pale cold skin	Pale cold skin
Shivering	No shivering	No shivering
Tachycardia	Bradycardia	Bradycardia
Hypertension	Hypotension	Hypotension
Tachypnoea	Bradypnoea	Hypoventilation
	Confused/combative	Stupor/coma
		Areflexic
		Oliguria
		Arrhythmias:
		AF
		Nodal/block
		VEs
		VF
		Asystole

Special considerations

ABC

A: With a fall in the consciousness level the cough and gag reflexes become impaired, thus aspiration pneumonia is more common.

B: As the core temperature falls there is a leftward shift in the oxy-haemoglobin dissociation curve, making oxygen release to tissues more difficult. However, hypothermia also reduces oxygen requirements.

C: A 'cold diuresis' with subsequent hypovolaemia can occur because of an impairment of renal concentrating ability. This is aggravated by a plasma shift into the extravascular space.

Caution is needed with regard to the rate of fluid administration because the cold myocardium does not tolerate excessive fluid loads.

With a progressive fall in core temperature sinus bradycardia gives way to atrial fibrillation with a slow ventricular response. Eventually ventricular fibrillation and ultimately asystole occur. Furthermore, in severe hypothermia the myocardium can became very sensitive to the mildest of stimuli, such as simply moving the patient. Thus inappropriate cardiac massage can precipitate ventricular fibrillation which is resistant to electrical therapy until the core temperature is elevated.

General

The immobile hypothermic patient is liable to develop rhabdomyolysis with acute tubular necrosis. Thrombosis can occur, with subsequent embolic complications.

Treatment of hypothermia

The treatment of hypothermia depends upon its cause, rate of onset, duration, the cardiovascular status of the patient and the facilities available.

In cardiac arrest it is essential to raise the 'core' (deep body) temperature as rapidly as possible, by all available means, to greater than 32°C. Below this temperature defibrillation is unlikely to succeed (the initial three shocks of the VF algorithm should be given but repeated attempts will cause myocardial damage and should therefore be avoided). Drug treatments are also usually ineffective. Spontaneous reversion to an effective rhythm may occur with elevation of deep body temperature to greater than 32°C.

Severe hypothermia in a patient with an effective rhythm carries a significant risk of life-threatening dysrhythmias and therefore rapid rewarming to 32°C is justified. Extreme care should be taken, however, to avoid precipitating such dysrhythmias by interventions aimed at effecting rapid rewarming.

A previously healthy patient with mild or moderate hypothermia will generally spontaneously rewarm with passive techniques. More active measures are indicated if there is failure to spontaneously rewarm at approximately 1°C/h or if the underlying cause, such as drug intoxication or previous medical illness, cannot be countered. As a rule of thumb, if the patient has got cold slowly they should be rewarmed slowly, and if the onset is rapid and the duration short then rapid rewarming can be considered.

Passive rewarming

This requires metabolic heat production greater than the heat loss for the patient. The patient must be removed from the hostile environment, dried if wet, stripped of wet clothing and insulated with blankets. Covering the head significantly reduces heat loss and should be considered to be essential even in a warm hospital. Careful monitoring of progress is vital.

Warmed fluids

Warm oral fluids (in the conscious patient) and warmed intravenous fluids will prevent adding further to heat loss, and may contribute a little to a positive heat balance. Caution is needed with intravenous fluids in order not to overload the cold myocardium. Very large fluid volumes would be required to contribute greatly to rewarming.

Warmed humidified inspired air

This should be used when available, but only contributes to insulation by minimizing respiratory heat loss. In itself it contributes little to rewarming.

Active external rewarming

Immersion up to the neck in stirred warm water (40°C) will effect rapid rewarming, but is appropriate only in conscious, uninjured patients with a deep body temperature of greater than 30°C. It should be reserved for short-duration hypothermia of rapid onset. When the hypothermia has developed slowly and has been prolonged, there is profound acidosis in under-perfused peripheral tissues and hypovolaemia due to cold diuresis (and hydrostatically elevated venous pressure in immersion). The rapid vasodilatation produced by active external rewarming in warm water may therefore result in 'post-rescue' circulatory collapse. If this method is used a significant 'afterdrop' in the measured deep body temperature (especially if measured rectally) may be seen. This is commonly attributed to a return of cold blood to the central circulation from the periphery; however, it has been proven experimentally that this is not the case and that there is no fall in central blood temperature. The phenomenon can be explained purely on the laws of physics and is seen to occur in the absence of any circulation. There is therefore little risk of lowering the cardiac temperature to arrhythmia thresholds. Circulating water blankets, electric blankets, warm air blankets, heating cradles, etc. will achieve the same effect as warm bath rewarming, but less efficiently; however, it may be useful when immersion in warm water is impractical. Care must be taken not to thermally injure the skin. There is no benefit to excluding the limbs as the perceived risks of a 'cold shock' to the heart are not a reality.

Active internal rewarming

This entails the active addition of heat directly to the 'core' by irrigation of hollow organs (stomach and bladder) and body cavities (pleura and peritoneum) with warm fluid (40°C). These techniques require varying degrees of expertise and equipment and are appropriate only in extreme conditions such as cardiac arrest. Irrigation fluids should be isotonic and potassium free. These interventions will effect rewarming but must be continued for prolonged periods, often several hours, to raise the temperature to greater than 32°C in severely hypothermic arrested patients. CPR may be required for extended periods and the facilities of an intensive care unit are recommended. Extracorporeal blood rewarming using haemodialysis equipment, haemofiltration equipment or cardiopulmonary bypass can effect rewarming very rapidly but has limited availability and requires very specialized skills and monitoring. These techniques should be considered in the potentially salvageable patient even if transfer to another facility would be required.

Basic life support

Measures should be taken to prevent any further heat loss if possible. The patient should be handled as gently as possible throughout, to prevent the stimulation of ventricular fibrillation in the sensitive myocardium.

ABC

C: The pulse should be felt for 60 s to ensure detection of the most severe bradycardia. Only if no pulse is detected should external cardiac massage be started.

Advanced life support

Patients who have a palpable output but are severely hypothermic should be handled as gently as possible, in order to reduce the risk of inducing a dysrhythmia.

ABC

C: Dysrhythmias tend to spontaneously correct themselves as the deep body temperature rises. In VF, after the initial three shocks and once a reliable deep body temperature has been established, further attempts at cardioversion should be avoided until the temperature exceeds 32°C.

General

The patient is not dead until both warm and dead. Life support measures must continue until a deep body temperature of at least 32°C has been achieved. Only then can a definite diagnosis of death be made.

Post-resuscitation care

A chest radiograph and a 12-lead ECG are both essential. The latter may show 'J' waves (best seen in the V leads). These can occur at any subnormal temperature and so have no prognostic power. The plasma electrolytes, alcohol, thyroid function, blood cultures, drug screen, glucose and ABG should be measured. The ABG analysis will need to be corrected for the low core temperature.

PREGNANCY

Incidence

Cardiac arrest occurs about once every 30 000 pregnancies.

Aetiology and mechanism

In addition to the usual causes amniotic fluid embolus, eclampsia, and uteroplacental haemorrhage may all result in cardiorespiratory arrest. Pulmonary embolus is more common.

Special considerations

In late pregnancy there are a number of anatomical and physiological changes which must be taken into account during attempted resuscitation.

ABC

A: The airway may be difficult to control due to neck obesity, breast enlargement and possible supraglottic oedema. There is an increased risk of regurgitation and subsequent aspiration, both because of pressure on the stomach from the gravid uterus and because of delayed gastric emptying.

B: Oxygen consumption is increased due to the metabolic demands of pregnancy, but chest compliance and functional residual capacity are decreased for mechanical reasons.

C: In the supine position the uterus compresses the inferior vena cava resulting in reduced venous return.

Basic life support

Since oxygen consumption is increased, the pregnant patient will develop cerebral hypoxia more rapidly than the non-pregnant. Basic life support should therefore be initiated as quickly as possible.

ABC

A: Cricoid pressure should be applied by an assistant while ventilating the patient. This will reduce the risk of aspiration of gastric contents.

C: Pressure on the inferior vena cava should be relieved so that venous return is increased, otherwise cardiac massage will not produce an adequate output. This can be achieved either by inclining the patient 30° laterally (using a wedge under the right side) (Figure 13.1) or by an assistant manually moving the uterus to the left and towards the head (Figure 13.2).

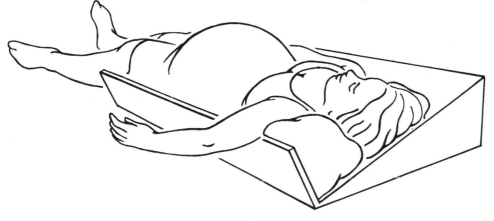

Figure 13.1 Lateral tilt using an obstetric wedge

Advanced life support

Any obvious causes of the arrest, such as hypovolaemia or status epilepticus secondary to eclampsia, should be treated.

ABC

A: Cricoid pressure should be maintained until the airway is both controlled and protected. Intubation is more difficult but should be attempted as soon as possible. It may prove impossible to insert a standard laryngoscope as the breasts can obstruct the handle. This problem can be overcome in one of two ways. Either a special laryngoscope is used or the blade of a standard laryngoscope is put in the mouth and the handle attached afterwards.

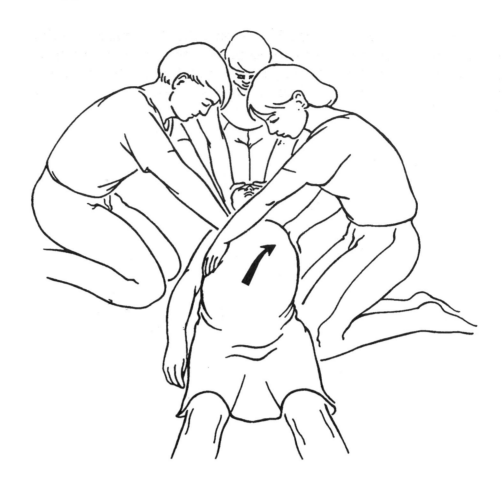

**Figure 13.2
Manual
displacement of
the uterus**

C: Dysrhythmias should be treated according to standard protocols unless the patient has undergone epidural anaesthesia. In that situation the following modifications to drug protocols apply:

1. Adrenaline should be administered early to counteract vasodilatation.
2. Lignocaine should be avoided as cumulation with the anaesthetic agent used for the epidural may prove toxic. Bretylium tosylate is therefore the preferred drug for the treatment of refractory VF in this situation.

General

If resuscitation is unsuccessful after 5 min then emergency caesarean section should be performed. This improves the mother's chances of survival as the inferior vena cava is further decompressed, and also helps the fetus. ACLS should continue throughout surgery.

Post-resuscitation care

Surviving patients will all require urgent obstetric consultation, and paediatricians should be called to look after the child. Specific obstetric causes of the arrest should be sought and treated appropriately. Since aspiration of acid gastric contents is likely, the resulting chemical pneumonitis (Mendelsohn's syndrome) should be sought and treated.

DRUG OVERDOSES

Aetiology and mechanism

Cardiovascular compromise or cardiorespiratory arrest may be caused by either an accidental or a deliberate drug overdose. In the older patient prescribed drugs are usually responsible, whereas in younger patients abuse of either prescribed or illegal drugs is seen. Alcohol is often a complicating factor. The identity of the abused substance must be ascertained as soon as possible, and the effects noted. This may allow appropriate treatment to be commenced early enough to prevent cardiac arrest. If arrest does occur, the usual treatment protocols may be inadequate.

Special considerations

ABC

A: Patients with an altered consciousness level may have an absent gag reflex, and therefore an inadequately protected airway.

B: Hypoxia potentiates the deleterious effects of any drug overdose which causes embarrassment of the cardiovascular system. Oxygen is therefore a key treatment.

General

Hypoglycaemia can occur after overdosage, especially if alcohol is also involved. Blood glucose must always be measured early and any abnormalities promptly treated.

Combined drug overdoses may be more difficult to treat, and larger than normal doses of pharmaceutical agents may be required to achieve a desired effect. Treatment should be aimed at prevention of cardiac arrest, so every effort must be made to increase drug elimination from the body. Methods include administration of ipecacuanha syrup as an emetic, and stomach washout. The use of charcoal is limited by its palatability, but it can be very effective in absorbing drugs.

Advanced life support

ABC

A: The gag reflex should be sought and the airway adequately protected if it is absent.

C: Apparent VF may in fact be torsade de pointes. All class Ia anti-arrhythmic drugs (which increase the duration of repolarization) predispose to torsade. In toxic dosage tricyclic antidepressants are another potential cause.

General

If indicated, the residual drug should be eliminated from the stomach by lavage, and from the gut by administering activated charcoal. Lavage may cause excess vagal activity due to oropharyngeal stimulation, especially in beta-blocker overdoses.

Specific drugs

Opiates

There is little hope of resuscitating an opiate overdose without the administration of large quantities of naloxone. An intravenous dose of 0.4–1.6 mg should be given initially; this should be repeated at regular intervals throughout the resuscitation period. The short half-life of naloxone requires that a continuous infusion be commenced when resuscitation is successful. An initial rate of 0.4–0.8 mg/h (in 5% dextrose) is used, and this is titrated to clinical effect. IM naloxone has a longer half-life, and may be of use in the non-co-operative addict. Naloxone will, of course, precipitate an acute withdrawal state in such addicts.

Beta-blockers

The most severe effects of beta-blocker overdose (pallor, hypotension, bradycardia and hypoglycaemia) are associated with the least cardioselective drugs such as propranolol. Patients may respond to the standard bradycardia protocol, but if they don't intravenous glucagon should be given. The dose in adults is 5–10 mg stat, followed by an infusion at 1–5 mg/h. In children the doses are 0.15 mg/kg and 0.05–0.1 mg/kg/h respectively.

Tricyclic antidepressants

This group of drugs is particularly dangerous. They induce a state of cardiac irritability which may result in the development of a variety of drug-resistant, and often life-threatening, dysrhythmias. These may develop or recur for up to 24–36 h after ingestion. A prolonged QT interval is associated with a higher incidence of dysrhythmias. Whatever the rhythm on the ECG, the initial treatment is 1–2 mmol/kg of sodium bicarbonate IV (50 ml 8.4% solution as an initial bolus for an adult). Even in VF, sodium bicarbonate should be given early – after the first three DC shocks. Further aliquots of 50 ml should be given until either the blood pH is 7.55 or the dysrhythmia has reverted to sinus rhythm. Tricyclics can also cause fits and hyperthermia, both of which should be treated in the usual way.

Washout is only for people who have a life-threatening overdose within 1–2 h of ingestion.

Cardiac glycosides

Acute poisoning with cardiac glycosides causes a raised serum potassium and conduction abnormalities (mostly varying degrees of A-V block). Chronic poisoning is often associated with a low or normal serum potassium and, unusually, serious dysrhythmias such as VT or VF may develop, apparently aggravated by the hypokalaemia.

Digoxin

Only about 20% of an oral dose is absorbed, and it takes 6–12 h before this is fixed in the tissues. If life-threatening dysrhythmias do occur they should be treated according to the usual protocols. In addition, digoxin-specific (Fab) antibodies should be given. It takes some 30–60 min for these to begin to reverse the signs of digoxin intoxication, and the peak effect is seen at 3 h. Each 40 mg of antibodies binds 0.6 mg of digoxin; consequently the dose required varies with the size of the overdose.

Digoxin-specific (Fab) antibodies are kept in regional and sub-regional centres only, but are available urgently on demand. Any poisons unit will be able to give the name of the nearest hospital that can supply them, and any contact names and numbers that are required.

TRAUMA

Aetiology and mechanism

Trauma can cause cardiac dysrhythmia or arrest in a number of ways. Direct injury to the heart may be so severe as to cause disruption (which is invariably fatal), cardiac tamponade or cardiac contusion with its attendant risks of dysrhythmias. Injuries to the chest can also precipitate a cardiac arrest secondary to hypoxia, or restriction of the mediastinum due to a tension pneumothorax. Finally, severe bleeding may cause hypovolaemic arrest. All of the treatable causes of traumatic cardiac dysrhythmia and arrest are dealt with elsewhere in this text, and are not dealt with again here. Reference may be found to them as follows:

- Hypoxia: Airway management (Chapter 6)

- Tension pneumothorax: Treatment protocols (Chapter 9)

- Cardiac contusion: Dysrhythmia management (Chapter 8)

- Cardiac tamponade: Treatment protocols (Chapter 9)

- Hypovolaemia: Treatment protocols (Chapter 9)

ELECTRICAL INJURIES

Aetiology and mechanism

Electrical injuries occur either because of contact with power sources, or because of lightning strike.

Power sources

Dry skin offers high resistance to electricity. However, skin that has been moistened with water, sweat, or other conductive fluid has a much reduced resistance. The injury caused depends on the nature and size of the current, the duration, the area exposed, and the path the current follows. DC is less dangerous than AC. AC currents of 25–300 Hz and 25–240 V tend to cause ventricular fibrillation if the path crosses the heart. If the voltage is over 1000 V respiratory paralysis is common. At intermediate currents a mixed picture of dysrhythmia with respiratory insufficiency is likely.

Lightning

Lightning is a direct current which travels from thunderclouds to the ground at speeds of up to 1 million metres per second. It can attain voltages of more than 100 million volts and temperatures of up to 3000°C. Lightning injuries may be from direct strikes, splash from surrounding structures, or step voltage (the transmission of ground surface current through a circuit created by the victim's legs).

Cardiac arrest may occur as the result of sudden cardiac standstill caused by the huge DC countershock of the lightning strike. Both ventricular fibrillation and asystole have been reported. Respiratory arrest is the most common cause of death following lightning strike, and may occur due to brain stem shock, contusion or because of respiratory muscle paralysis. Respiratory arrest can be complicated by cardiac arrest either because of simultaneous cardiac standstill or secondary hypoxic effects. Myocardial infarction may occur as an acute complication.

Special considerations

In the case of injury from power sources, diagnosis is usually from the history. If lightning strike has occurred, and no history is available, characteristic 'flashover' burn injury patterns may aid diagnosis:

1. **Linear:** Superficial and partial thickness, beginning at the head and neck, and flowing in a branching pattern down the chest and legs.
2. **Feathering:** These are the cutaneous imprints of electron showers. They appear like a delicately branching fern.
3. **Punctate:** Full or partial thickness, circular in clusters that form star-burst patterns.

Safety

Electrical current can cause continued injury to the patient, and significant injury to the rescuer.

ABC

A: Electrical burns to the face and airway may occur.

Basic life support

SAFE

The victim should be freed from the current at once by turning off the power.

It is essential that all danger to the rescuer and rescue area should be minimized first

Advanced life support

ABC

A: If facial burns have occurred intubation may be difficult. It is important to achieve definitive airway care early, as difficulty will increase with time. Specialist anaesthetic help should be sought in this situation, and surgical control of the airway may be necessary.

Post-resuscitation care

If resuscitation is successful (return of spontaneous circulation) the patient should be maintained on a ventilator for 12–24 h before weaning is attempted. This is to allow time for spontaneous respiratory activity to return. Cardiac monitoring should continue throughout this period. Fixed dilated pupils are of no prognostic significance following electrical injury.

SMOKE INHALATION

Aetiology and mechanism

Smoke inhalation may cause three types of injury:

1. Thermal injury to the airways.
2. Chemical injury to the airways and lungs.
3. Systemic poisoning.

Agents involved in chemical injury include acrolein (a highly reactive aldehyde) from wood and petroleum products, hydrochloric acid from polyvinyl chloride, toluene diisocyanate from polyurethane, and nitrogen dioxide from cars and agricultural wastes. Carbon monoxide formed during incomplete combustion, and cyanide found during house fires, both cause systemic poisoning.

A combination of thermal injury and poisoning, together with lowering of inspired oxygen levels during the fire, can result in hypoxic cardiorespiratory arrest.

Special considerations

All patients presenting following a fire in an enclosed space should be suspected of suffering from smoke injury. Carbonaceous sputum and perioral burns also strongly suggest this diagnosis.

Safety

Continued exposure to smoke can continue to cause injury to the patient and can harm the rescuer.

ABC

A: Airway management may be complicated by perioral burns and thermal burns to the airways themselves.

B: Carbon monoxide poisoning may occur. The high affinity of carboxyhaemoglobin for oxygen further exacerbates tissue hypoxia. Carboxyhaemoglobin levels will start to decrease once the victim is removed from the toxic environment, even if they are breathing air, and this should be borne in mind. Immediate estimations should be interpreted as shown in Table 13.4.

Table 13.4 Immediate estimations of carboxyhaemoglobin level

	Carboxyhaemoglobin level
Non-smokers	<1%
Smokers	4–6%
Significant exposure	>10%

The use of a pulse oximeter will be falsely reassuring, because only normal saturated haemoglobin will be measured. At carboxyhaemoglobin levels above 50% myocardial infarction may occur, especially in individuals with pre-existing ischaemic disease. Alkalosis and hypothermia decrease the dissociation of carbon monoxide and should be avoided.

Basic life support

SAFE

The victim should be removed from the smoke-filled environment as soon as possible. It may be necessary for a rescuer wearing breathing apparatus to do this.

Advanced life support

ABC

A: If peri-oral, neck or airway burns have occurred intubation may be difficult. It is important to achieve definitive airway care early, as difficulty will increase with time. Specialist anaesthetic help should be sought in this situation, and surgical control of the airway may be necessary.

B: Urgent estimation of carboxyhaemoglobin levels should be undertaken. Care must be taken not to cause respiratory alkalosis by hyperventilation.

General

Hypothermia should be corrected as discussed in the relevant section.

Post-resuscitation care

If spontaneous respiration returns and carbon monoxide levels are not raised, close monitoring for late-onset bronchospasm and pulmonary oedema is required. This may occur up to 24 h after exposure. If carbon monoxide levels are significantly raised, ventilation with 100% oxygen should be continued at least until levels are within the normal range. The use of hyperbaric oxygen is preferred, as this reduces the time taken for the restoration of normal haemoglobin. Local specialist advice is therefore required.

VOLATILE SUBSTANCE ABUSE

Incidence and aetiology

The incidence of deaths from the inhalation of volatile substances in the UK is significant – 856 deaths between 1981 and 1989. Most abusers are between 10 and 18 years of age.

A wide variety of readily available volatile substances may be abused in this way: many glues contain toluene, cleaning fluids contain trichloroethylene or other chlorinated hydrocarbons, propellants for aerosols (chlorofluorocarbons), gases like propane and butane, standard fuels such as petrol and paraffin.

Special considerations

A substance entering the body by inhalation delivers a high concentration to the brain quickly, giving the patient a 'rush' or 'buzz'. Early symptoms are similar to those of alcohol intoxication. Patients may be aggressive towards others or may harm themselves. The initial euphoria, blurred vision and feelings of omnipotence give way to loss of consciousness if inhalation is continued. Volatile substance abuse is usually a group activity. When one person becomes unconscious, the others wait for spontaneous recovery. When this does not happen, there is an inevitable delay before help is summoned, which prejudices the chances of a successful resuscitation.

Basic life support

SAFE

Volatile substances are inflammable. There may be a strong concentration of substances in the rescue area which could affect the rescuer. There is also a small risk of contamination by mouth to mouth or mouth to nose ventilation.

ABC

A: The feeling of power and sensation of being able to fly induced by volatile substances sometimes leads a person to take risks, which result in serious injury. If the situation indicates a possibility of injury to the patient as well as the direct toxic effects of the abused substance, the airway should be managed in conjunction with in-line cervical spine immobilization. The airway is at risk because early central nervous system excitation causes vomiting. This is compounded by later effects which impair the level of consciousness. Convulsions are yet another possible cause of airway embarrassment.

B: Breathing can be compromised early on by bronchospasm, which is treated as usual with bronchodilators. Later, respiratory depression is marked. Respiratory support is essential where the patient is unconscious.

Advanced life support

ABC

A: Definitive airway management is by endotracheal intubation, but the cervical spine must be protected throughout the procedure.

B: Depression of the central nervous system is one of the mechanisms leading to death. Delivery of high-flow oxygen with full ventilatory support is essential. Inhalation of amyl or butyl nitrites leads to severe or life-threatening methaemoglobinaemia. This clinical picture is a hypoxic patient, with slate-grey skin colour, who does not respond to increasing concentrations of inspired oxygen. The patient's blood is 'chocolate brown' in colour. Treatment with IV methylene blue is required.

C: The circulation is jeopardized during volatile substance abuse by arrhythmias. Cardiac arrest can occur as asystole, as the end result of a severe bradycardia, or in ventricular fibrillation. It is likely that the myocardium becomes sensitized to endogenous catecholamines. It has been shown that adrenaline and asphyxia increase

the arrhythmogenic potential of solvents, and that ethanol can further predispose to cardiac irregularity. Studies have also demonstrated that this sensitivity persists for several hours after inhalant exposure (unlike the CNS depressant effects, which are short-lived).

The risk of sudden death is higher if propellants or butane are sprayed directly down the throat. The sudden cooling of the throat and larynx causes a severe vagal inhibition reflex, with marked cardiac slowing/standstill.

Post-resuscitation care

The volatile properties of abused substances ensure that they are rapidly excreted from the lungs; thus the CNS depressant effects are short-lived. Once the patient is conscious and breathing adequately, he usually absconds from further care. However, he is still at risk of developing potentially fatal arrhythmias for several hours from myocardial sensitization to endogenous catecholamines.

ANAPHYLAXIS

Allergic reactions (mostly IgE mediated) can be sudden and severe. Dermal contact with an allergen results in weals, erythematous skin and watering, itchy eyes. However, when the allergen is introduced directly into the body by inhalation, injection, bites or stings, the reaction in sensitized individuals tends to be rapid and severe. It may be life-threatening if untreated. Anaphylaxis is more common than once supposed. It can occur without warning in an individual who has been exposed to the same antigen on previous occasions without adverse effects.

Basic life support

SAFE

A substance which causes anaphylaxis in one individual is unlikely to do so in another, so there should not be an immediate risk to the rescuer.

ABC

A: Rapid development of angio-oedema and laryngeal oedema results in early airway compromise. The usual airway-opening manoeuvres will probably be ineffective. The patient will be distressed, with noisy breathing, and will want to sit up initially.

Nausea and vomiting are common, further putting the airway at risk.

B: Respiratory distress may be compounded by the development of bronchospasm. It is essential to get help so that the patient can receive advanced life support as soon as possible. If oxygen is available, this should be given in the highest concentration possible.

C: When a specific antigen meets a specific immunoglobulin (IgE) bound to mast cells and basophils it triggers the release of histamine and other vasoactive substances. These cause both vasodilatation and an increase in vascular permeability. Tachycardia and hypotension develop as a result of the increased vascular space available and because fluid is lost from the circulation.

Anaphylactoid reactions also occur, e.g. after administration of blood products or iodinated contrast media. These have the same vascular effects but do not involve prior sensitization or mediation through IgE.

Treatment is urgent. Help must be obtained quickly so that advanced life support measures can be given.

Advanced life support

ABC

A: High-flow oxygen must be given via the most suitable delivery system for the condition of the patient. If stridor is present or if the patient has difficulty maintaining their airway, endotracheal intubation is necessary. Ideally, this should be carried out only by a highly experienced operator. Intubation will be complicated by laryngeal oedema and intraoral swelling. The tongue may be considerably enlarged. If endo- or nasotracheal intubation are not possible and the patient continues to deteriorate, a surgical airway must be performed immediately, by needle cricothyroidotomy or surgical cricothyroidotomy.

B: Delivery of high-flow oxygen to the lungs may not ensure adequate oxygenation. Bronchospasm and pulmonary oedema can make ventilation difficult, even with positive pressure. Bronchospasm should be treated vigorously with nebulized bronchodilators and, when IV access has been achieved, with IV hydrocortisone.

C: Hypotension will be refractory and progress to cardiac arrest if not treated vigorously with intravenous fluids and IM or IV adrenaline. Any IV fluid will be satisfactory, as long as enough is given, although colloid is preferable. Adrenaline should be given as soon as possible. If the patient still has a cardiac output either 1:1000, 0.5–1 mg (0.5–1.0 ml) IM or 1:10 000, 0.1–0.2 (1–2 ml) IV should suffice. An antihistamine, such as Chlorpheniramine 10 mg, should also be given IV.

If the patient has arrested, the usual protocols should be followed but adrenaline 1:10 000 1 mg (10 ml) should be given as soon as possible.

Once a patient has deteriorated to cardiac arrest, successful resuscitation is difficult. It is essential to recognize the potential problems early and treat them aggressively.

Post-resuscitation care

If the patient has not yet arrested, the airway has been secured and blood pressure controlled with adrenaline, the patient will survive this episode. However, they should be admitted to hospital and monitored in a high-dependency environment. Minor hypotensive relapses and recurrences of bronchospasm still require early recognition and treatment.

On restoration of cardiac output after cardiorespiratory arrest, the patient should be admitted to intensive care facilities. Ventilation should continue until laryngeal oedema, tongue swelling and bronchospasm have all settled. The heart rate and blood pressure must be continuously monitored and small incremental doses of IV adrenaline 1:10 000 given (e.g. 0.3–0.5 mg or 3–5 ml over 5 min), titrating them against the patient's response. Vomiting, abdominal pain and diarrhoea usually settle down over 2–3 h. On recovery and discharge, the patient must be appraised of the risks if the same antigen is encountered again, and the importance of carrying an adrenaline pen for self-injection emphasized.

SUMMARY

Most cardiac arrests can be dealt with satisfactorily by reference to the standard protocols. This chapter has outlined those conditions which are associated with cardiac arrest where to achieve optimal outcome, significant changes are required. However, the ABC system still takes priority, whatever the cause of the cardiac arrest.

SECTION FOUR
Practical procedures

14

Procedures – airway control and ventilation

Procedures

- Oropharyngeal airway insertion
- Nasopharyngeal airway insertion
- Ventilation via a Laerdal Pocket Mask
- Orotracheal intubation: adult; paediatric
- Insertion of a laryngeal mask airway
- Insertion of a Combitube
- Surgical airway: needle cricothyroidotomy; surgical cricothyroidotomy

---

OROPHARYNGEAL AIRWAY

Having chosen one of the correct size by comparing the airway with the distance from the angle of the jaw to the corner of the mouth, the technique used for insertion in adults and older children is as follows:

1. The patient's mouth is opened and a check made for debris that may be pushed into the larynx as the airway is inserted.
2. The airway is inserted into the mouth 'upside down' (concave uppermost) as far as the junction between hard and soft palates.
3. It is then rotated through 180°.
4. It is now fully inserted so that the flange lies in front of the upper and lower incisors or gums in the edentulous patient (Figure 14.1).
5. After insertion, check the patency of airway and ventilation by 'looking, listening and feeling'.

In infants and small children the correct size is estimated using the vertical distance from the angle of the jaw or tragus to the corner of the mouth. To insert the airway:

1. The mouth is opened.
2. A tongue depressor or the tip of a laryngoscope blade is used to aid insertion of the airway 'the right way up' under direct vision.

**Figure 14.1
Oropharyngeal
airway *in situ***

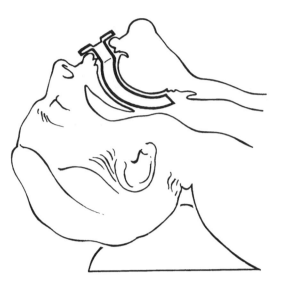

The soft palate is easily damaged if the airway is inserted using the adult technique.

Complications

- Airway obstruction is worsened.

- Trauma, causing bleeding.

- Vomiting or laryngospasm if the patient is not deeply unconscious.

NASOPHARYNGEAL AIRWAY

Use with caution if there is a suspected fracture to the base of the skull.

Choose an airway approximately the same size as the patient's little finger or similar in diameter to the nares. Airways are designed to be inserted with the bevel facing medially; consequently the right nostril is usually tried first, using the following technique:

1. The airway is thoroughly lubricated.
2. The patency of the right nostril is checked.
3. The airway is inserted, bevel end first, along the floor of the nose (i.e. vertically in a supine patient) with a gentle twisting action.
4. When fully inserted, the flange should lie at the nares (Figure 14.2).
5. Once the airway is in place, a safety-pin can be inserted through the flange to prevent the airway being inhaled.
6. If the right nostril is occluded or obstruction to insertion is met, the left nostril should be used.
7. After insertion, check patency of the airway and ventilation by 'looking, listening and feeling'.

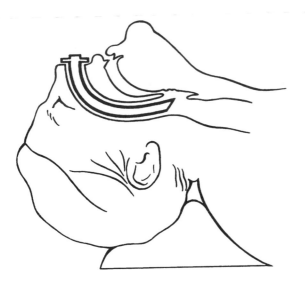

**Figure 14.2
Nasopharyngeal
airway *in situ***

Complications

- Bleeding.
- Vomiting and laryngospasm if the patient is not deeply unconscious.

LAERDAL POCKET MASK

The technique for using the mask is as follows:

1. With the patient supine, the mask is applied to the face using the thumbs and index fingers of both hands.
2. The remaining fingers are used to exert pressure behind the angles of the jaw (as for jaw thrust) at the same time as the mask is pressed onto the face to make a tight seal (Figure 14.3).

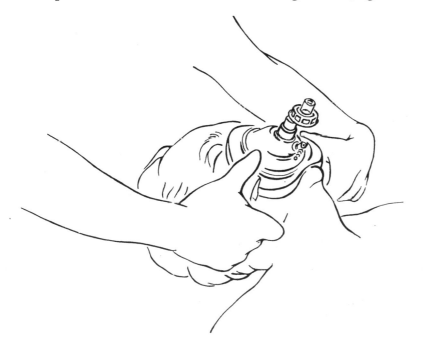

**Figure 14.3
Mouth to mask
ventilation**

3. The rescuer then blows through the inspiratory valve for 1–2 s, at the same time watching to ensure the chest rises and then falls.
4. If oxygen is available it should be added via the nipple at 4–6 l/min.

OROTRACHEAL INTUBATION

Orotracheal intubation in adults and older children

Box 14.1   Equipment for orotracheal intubation in adults

1. Laryngoscope: most commonly with a curved (Macintosh) blade
2. Tracheal tubes: females 7.5–8.0 mm internal diameter, 21 cm long; males 8.0–9.0 mm internal diameter, 23 cm long
3. Syringe, to inflate the cuff
4. Catheter mount, to attach to ventilating device
5. Lubricant for tube; water soluble, preferably sterile
6. Magills forceps
7. Introducers, malleable and gum elastic, for difficult cases
8. Adhesive tapes or bandages for securing tube
9. Ventilator
10. Suction

1. Whenever possible, intubation should be preceded by a period of ventilation with 100% oxygen, using a bag-valve-mask device. During this time, the equipment to be used must be checked for completeness and function, particularly the laryngoscope, suction and ventilating device.
2. Choose a tracheal tube of the appropriate length and diameter and check the integrity of the cuff.
3. Position the patient's head to facilitate intubation; flex the neck and extend the head at the atlantooccipital joint (the 'sniffing the morning air' position). This is often made easier by placing a small pillow under the patient's head.
4. Holding the laryngoscope in the left hand, open the patient's mouth and introduce the blade into the right-hand side of the mouth, displacing the tongue to the left.
5. Pass the blade along the edge of the tongue; the tip of the epiglottis should be seen emerging at the base of the tongue.
6. Advance the tip of the blade between the base of the tongue and the anterior surface of the epiglottis (vallecula).

7. The tongue and epiglottis are then **lifted** to reveal the vocal cords. Note that **the laryngoscope must be lifted in the direction that the handle is pointing and not levered** by movement of the wrist, as this might damage the teeth and will not provide as good a view (Figure 14.4).

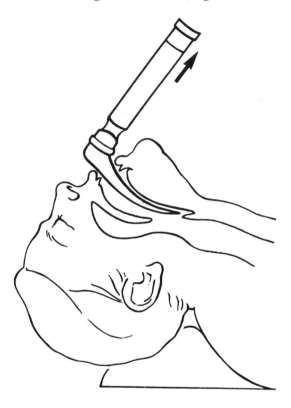

**Figure 14.4
Direct
laryngoscopy**

8. Introduce the tracheal tube from the right-hand side of the mouth and insert it between the vocal cords into the larynx under direct vision, until the cuff just passes the cords.
9. Once the tube is in place, inflate the cuff sufficiently to provide an airtight seal between the tube and the trachea. As an initial approximation, the same volume of air (in ml) can be used as the diameter of the tube in mm, and adjusted later.
10. A catheter mount is then attached to the tube and ventilation commenced.

Checks should then be made to ensure correct positioning of the tube and confirm ventilation of both lungs, by:

● Looking for bilateral chest movement with ventilation.

● Listening for breath sounds bilaterally in the mid-axillary line.

● Listening for gurgling sounds over the epigastrium, which may indicate inadvertent oesophageal intubation.

● Measurement of carbon dioxide in 'expired' gas. This will be >0.2% in gas leaving the lungs, providing there is a spontaneous circulation or good CPR is in progress. Less than 0.2% is strongly suggestive of oesophageal placement of the tube.

Complications

- All the structures encountered from the lips to the trachea may be traumatized.

- If the degree of unconsciousness has been misjudged, vomiting may be stimulated.

- The use of a tube that is too long may result in it passing into a main bronchus (usually the right), causing the opposite lung to collapse, and severely impairing the efficiency of ventilation. This is usually identified by the absence of breath sounds and reduced movement on the unventilated side.

- The most dangerous complication associated with tracheal intubation is **unrecognized oesophageal intubation**. The patient may appear to be ventilating adequately, but in fact is receiving no oxygen at all and rapidly becoming hypoxic. If in doubt, take it out and ventilate the patient using a bag-valve-mask.

Manoeuvres to assist with intubation

Occasionally, when the larynx is very anterior, direct pressure on the thyroid cartilage by an assistant may aid visualization of the vocal cords (not to be confused with cricoid pressure). However, despite this manoeuvre, in a small percentage of patients only the very posterior part of the cords (or none) can be seen and passage of the tracheal tube becomes difficult. In these cases, it is often possible to insert a gum-elastic introducer into the larynx initially and the tracheal tube slid over the introducer into the larynx. However, it must be remembered that the patient must be oxygenated between attempts at intubation.

Infants and small children

1. Whenever possible, intubation should be preceded by a period of ventilation with 100% oxygen, using a bag-valve-mask device. During this time, the equipment to be used must be checked for completeness and function, particularly the laryngoscope, suction and ventilating device.
2. Choose a tracheal tube of the correct length and diameter. Have available tubes a size above and below the best estimate.
3. Position the patient's head to facilitate intubation. In small babies, because of their relatively large occiput, it may be helpful to place a folded sheet under the back and neck to allow extension of the head.

Box 14.2   Equipment for orotracheal intubation in children

1. Laryngoscope: choice of straight blade (e.g. Miller, Seward) or curved blade (Macintosh)
2. Tracheal tubes: for children over 1 year size calculated from:

   internal diameter (mm) = age in years/4 + 4

   length (cm) = age in years/2 + 12

   1 month to 1 year, 3–3.5 mm diameter, 12 cm in length
   - One tube 0.5 mm smaller than calculated
   - One tube 5 mm larger than calculated
   - Uncuffed tubes in children under 8 years
3. Catheter mount, to attach to ventilating device
4. Lubricant
5. Magills forceps
6. Introducer
7. Adhesive tape for securing tube
8. Ventilator
9. Suction

4. Holding the laryngoscope with the left hand, open the patient's mouth and introduce the blade into the right-hand side of the mouth, displacing the tongue to the left.
5. The straight-bladed laryngoscope is often used in children under 6 months of age, and is designed to 'pick-up' the epiglottis. The tip of the blade is passed beyond the epiglottis into the upper oesophagus. The blade is then slowly withdrawn until the cords come into view. Once past 6 months a curved blade is used, as in the adult.
6. The tracheal tube is inserted from the right-hand side of the mouth into the larynx under direct vision. The tip should lie 2–4 cm beyond the vocal cords, depending on age. Most modern disposable tubes have a marker to indicate the length to place.
7. Check placement of the tube by:
   - looking for bilateral chest movement with ventilation
   - listening for breath sounds bilaterally in the mid-axillary line
   - listening for gurgling sounds over the epigastrium, which may indicate inadvertent oesophageal intubation
8. If intubation is not accomplished in less than 30 s, reestablish ventilation using a bag-valve-mask.

Insertion of the laryngeal mask airway

Box 14.3   Equipment for insertion of a laryngeal mask airway

1. Laryngeal mask airway size	Cuff volume (ml)
5 (large adult)	40
4 (adult male)	30
3 (adult female, child 30–35 kg)	20
2.5 (child, 15–30 kg)	15
2 (small child/infant)	10
1 (neonate/infant to 6.5 kg)	2–4

2. Lubricant
3. Syringe to inflate cuff
4. Adhesive tape to secure airway
5. Suction
6. Ventilating device

1. Whenever possible, insertion should be preceded by a period of ventilation with 100% oxygen, using a bag-valve-mask device. During this time, the equipment to be used must be checked for completeness and function, particularly the integrity of the cuff.
2. The cuff is deflated and the back and sides of the mask are lightly lubricated.
3. The patient's head is tilted (if safe to do so), the mouth opened fully and the tip of the mask inserted along the hard palate with the open side facing, but not touching the tongue (Figure 14.5a).
4. The mask is further inserted, along the posterior pharyngeal wall, with the operator's index finger initially providing support for the tube (Figure 14.5b). Eventually resistance is felt as the tip of the airway lies at the upper end of the oesophagus (Figure 14.5c).
5. The cuff is now fully inflated using the air-filled syringe attached to the valve at the end of the pilot tube using the volume of air shown in Box 14.3 (Figure 14.5d).
6. The airway is secured with adhesive tape and its position checked during ventilation as for a tracheal tube.
7. If insertion is not accomplished in under 30 s, re-establish ventilation using a bag-valve-mask.

Complications

- Incorrect placement, usually secondary to the tip of the cuff folding over during insertion. The airway should be withdrawn and reinserted.

- Inability to ventilate the patient due to displacement of the epiglottis over the larynx. Withdraw the airway and reinsert ensuring it follows closely the hard palate. This may be facili-

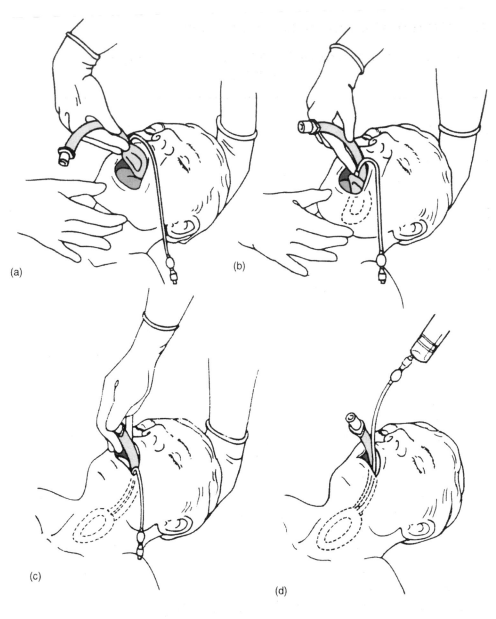
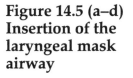

**Figure 14.5 (a–d)
Insertion of the
laryngeal mask
airway**

tated by the operator or an assistant lifting the jaw upwards.
Occasionally inability to insert may be due to rotation of the airway on insertion. Check that the line along the tube is aligned
with the patient's nasal septum; if not, reinsert.

● Coughing or laryngeal spasm, usually due to attempts to insert the
airway into a patient whose laryngeal reflexes are still present.

Intubation via the laryngeal mask airway

This can be achieved by inserting an introducer through the airway
into the trachea, removing the airway and then passing the tracheal
tube over the introducer into the trachea. Alternatively, a small-
diameter cuffed tracheal tube (6.0 mm) may be passed directly
through a size 4 or 5 LMA into the trachea. One specifically
designed to allow intubation through it, with a larger diameter tracheal tube, is currently being developed.

Insertion of a Combitube

Box 14.4   Equipment required for insertion of a Combitube

1. 37 or 41 FG Combitube
2. Accompanying syringes, 20 ml and 140 ml
3. Lubricant
4. Suction
5. Ventilating device

1. Whenever possible, insertion of a Combitube should be preceded by a period of ventilation with 100% oxygen, using a bag-valve-mask device. During this time, the equipment to be used must be checked for completeness and function, particularly the integrity of the cuffs.
2. The operator grasps the patient's jaw and tongue between thumb and index finger and lifts them forwards.
3. The tube is advanced with the curve pointing towards the larynx, in the midline, until the two black lines are positioned between the patient's teeth, or gums if edentulous.
4. The proximal cuff is inflated with 100 ml of air via the blue pilot tube marked 'No. 1'. The distal cuff is then inflated with 15 ml of air via the white pilot tube marked 'No. 2'.
5. Ventilation commences assuming oesophageal placement as this is the most common. The ventilating device is attached to the No. 1 (blue) end of the Combitube (Figure 14. 6a).
6. Confirmation that ventilation is successful (i.e. the Combitube lies in the oesophagus) as for placement of a tracheal tube.
7. If ventilation of the lungs is unsuccessful and accompanied by evidence of gastric inflation, the Combitube has passed into the trachea. The ventilating device should be connected to the No. 2 (clear, shorter) end of the Combitube (Figure 14.6b).
8. Confirm satisfactory ventilation as previously described.

In the oesophageal position regurgitation and aspiration is prevented by the distal cuff sealing the oesophagus. In the tracheal position aspiration of regurgitated contents is prevented by the distal cuff sealing the airway as with a conventional tracheal tube.

Complications

- Damage to the cuffs by the patient's teeth during insertion.
- Inability to insert due to limited mouth opening.
- Trauma to the oesophagus or trachea due to poor technique of insertion or wrong size used.
- Failure to achieve ventilation as a result of using the wrong lumen.

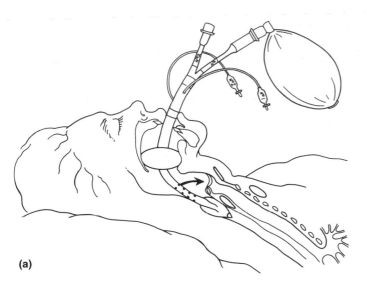

(a)

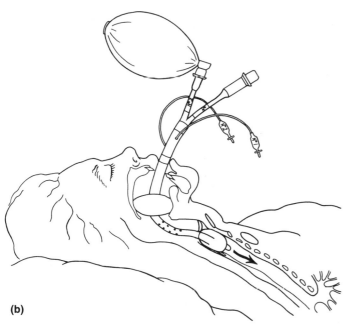

(b)

**Figure 14.6
Insertion of a
Combitube.
(a) Oesophageal
placement; (b)
tracheal
placement**

SURGICAL AIRWAY

It is important to realize that these techniques are temporizing measures, while preparations are being made to provide a definitive airway.

Needle cricothyroidotomy

1. The patient is placed supine with the head slightly extended.
2. The cricothyroid membrane is identified as the recess between the thyroid cartilage ('Adam's apple') and cricoid cartilage (approximately 2 cm below the 'V'-shaped notch of the thyroid cartilage).
3. This membrane is punctured vertically using a large-bore (12–14 g) intravenous cannula attached to a syringe.

4. Aspiration of air confirms that the tip of the cannula lies within the tracheal lumen.
5. The cannula is then angled at 45° caudally and advanced over the needle into the trachea (Figure 14.7).
6. The cannula is then attached to an oxygen supply at 12–15 l/min either via a 'Y' connector or through a hole cut in the side of the oxygen tubing. Oxygen is delivered by occluding the open limb of the connector or side hole for 1 s and then releasing for 4 s.
7. Expiration occurs passively through the larynx. The chest should be observed for movement and auscultated for breath sounds, although the latter are difficult to hear.
8. If satisfactorily placed, the cannula should be secured in place to prevent it being dislodged.

An alternative method of delivering oxygen is to use jet ventilation. This involves connecting the cannula to a high-pressure oxygen source (4 Bar, 400 kPa, 60 p.s.i.) via luer-lock connectors or by using a Sanders injector. The same ventilatory cycle is used.

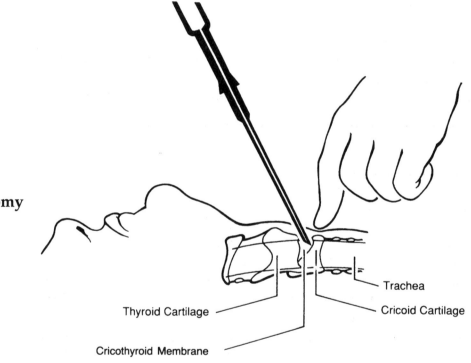

**Figure 14.7
Needle
cricothyroidotomy**

Trachea

Thyroid Cartilage

Cricoid Cartilage

Cricothyroid Membrane

Complications

- Asphyxia
- Pulmonary barotrauma
- Bleeding
- Oesophageal perforation
- Kinking of the cannula
- Surgical and mediastinal emphysema
- Aspiration

Occasionally, this method of oxygenation will disimpact a foreign body from the larynx, allowing resumption of more acceptable methods of ventilation.

> There are two important facts to remember about transtracheal insufflation of oxygen.
>
> First it is not possible to deliver oxygen via a needle cricothyroidotomy using a self-inflating bag and valve. This is because these devices do not generate sufficient pressure to drive adequate volumes of gas through a narrow cannula. In comparison, the wall oxygen supply will provide a pressure of 400 kPa (approximately 4000 cm H_2O), which overcomes the resistance of the cannula.
>
> Secondly, expiration cannot occur through the cannula, or through a separate cannula inserted through the cricothyroid membrane. The pressure generated during expiration is generally less than 3 kPa (30 cm H_2O), which is clearly much less than the pressure required to drive gas in initially. Expiration must occur through the upper airway, even when it is partially obstructed. If the obstruction is complete, then the oxygen flow must be reduced to 2–4 l/min to avoid the risk of barotrauma, in particular the creation of tension pneumothorax.

Surgical cricothyroidotomy

1. The patient is placed supine if possible with the head extended.
2. The cricothyroid membrane is identified as described above.
3. The thyroid cartilage is then stabilized using the thumb, index and middle fingers of the left hand.
4. If the patient is conscious, infiltration with local anaesthetic containing adrenaline (lignocaine 1% with adrenaline 1:80 000) should be considered.
5. A longitudinal incision is made down to the membrane, pressing the lateral edges of the skin outwards to reduce bleeding.
6. The membrane is incised transversely and the channel dilated with the scalpel handle to accept a small (4.0–7.0 mm) cuffed tracheostomy tube. If one of these is not immediately available, a similarly sized tracheal tube can be used.
7. The tube must enter the tracheal lumen, rather than just running anteriorly in the soft tissues.
8. The cuff is inflated and ventilation commenced.
9. Adequacy of ventilation must be checked by observation and auscultation of the chest and if satisfactory, the tube can be secured.
10. Suction is applied to the upper airway via tube to remove any inhaled blood or vomit.

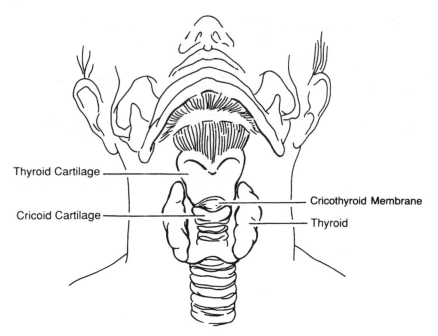

**Figure 14.8
Cricothyroidotomy
– relevant anatomy**

Thyroid Cartilage

Cricoid Cartilage

Cricothyroid Membrane

Thyroid

An alternative technique in these circumstances is the 'Mini-Trach' (Portex). Originally designed to facilitate the removal of secretions from the chest, this kit contains everything required to create an emergency surgical airway.

1. A guarded scalpel is used to puncture the cricothyroid membrane percutaneously, to the correct depth.
2. A rigid, curved introducer is then passed through the puncture site into the trachea.
3. A 4.0 mm PVC flanged tracheal cannula (with a standard 15 mm connector attached) is passed over the introducer into the trachea.
4. The introducer is then removed and the cannula secured with tapes via the flanges. The patient may then be ventilated using the devices already described.

Complications

Complications of performing a surgical airway are similar to those of needle cricothyroidotomy, except that bleeding is more profuse due to the larger incision. In the long term, damage to the vocal cords may result in hoarseness, and cricoid cartilage damage may cause laryngeal stenosis.

15
Practical procedures – access to the circulation

Procedures

- Peripheral venous cannulation
- Surgical cutdown
- Central venous cannulation: internal jugular vein; subclavian vein
- Intraosseous access

PERIPHERAL VENOUS CANNULATION

1. Choose a vein capable of accommodating a large cannula, preferably one that is both visible and palpable. The junction of two veins is often a good site as the 'target' is relatively larger.
2. Encourage the vein to dilate as this increases the success rate of cannulation. In the limb veins this is usually achieved by using a tourniquet which stops venous return from the limb but which permits arterial flow into the limb. Further dilatation can be encouraged by gently tapping the skin over the vein. In the patient who is cold and vasoconstricted, if time permits, topical application of heat from a towel soaked in warm water can also be useful.
3. If time permits the skin over the vein should now be cleaned. Ensure there is no risk of allergy if iodine-based agents are used. If alcohol-based agents are used, they must be given time to work (2–3 min), ensuring that the skin is dry before proceeding further.
4. In the conscious patient, consider infiltrating a small amount of local anaesthetic into the skin at the point chosen using a 22–25 g needle, particularly if a large (>1.2 mm, 18 g) cannula is to be used. This not only reduces the pain of cannulation, therefore making the patient less likely to move, but also makes them less resistant to further attempts if the first is unsuccessful!
5. If a large cannula is used, insertion through the skin may be facilitated by first making a small incision with either a 19 g needle or a scalpel blade, taking care not to puncture the vein.

6. The vein should now be immobilized to prevent it being displaced by the advancing cannula. This is achieved by pulling the skin over the vein tight with the spare hand (Figure 15.1).

**Figure 15.1
Vein
immobilized**

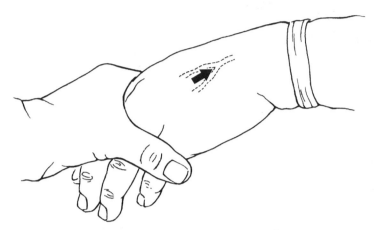

7. Holding the cannula firmly, at an angle of 10–15° to the skin, advance it through the skin and then into the vein. Often a slight loss of resistance is felt as the vein is entered. This should be accompanied by the appearance of blood in the flashback chamber of the cannula (Figure 15.2). However, the appearance of blood indicates only that the tip of the needle, not necessarily any of the cannula, is within the vein.

**Figure 15.2
Cannula
inserted: note
the flashback of
blood**

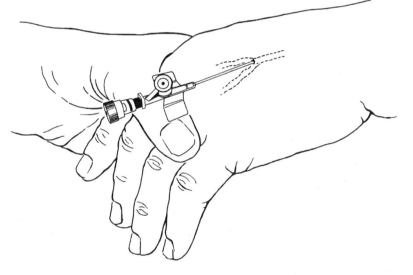

8. Keeping the skin taught, the next step is to reduce the angle of the cannula slightly and advance it a further 2–3 mm into the vein to ensure that the first part of the plastic cannula lies within the vein. Care must be taken at this point not to push the needle out of the back of the vein.
9. The needle is now withdrawn 5–10 mm into the cannula so that the point no longer protrudes from the end. Often, as this is done blood will be seen to flow between the needle body and the cannula, confirming that the tip of the cannula is within the vein (Figure 15.3).

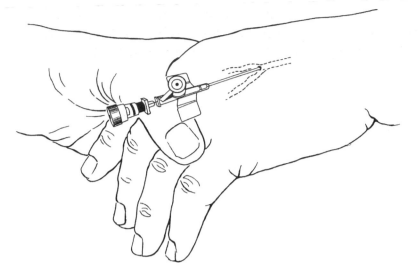

**Figure 15.3
Cannula with
needle slightly
withdrawn**

10. The cannula and needle combined should now be advanced along the vein. The needle is retained within the cannula to provide support and to prevent kinking at the point of skin puncture (Figure 15.4).

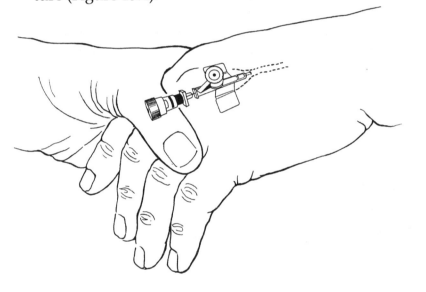

**Figure 15.4
Cannula fully
inserted**

11. Once the cannula is inserted as far as the hub, the tourniquet should be released and the needle completely removed and disposed of safely.
12. Confirmation that the cannula lies within the vein should be made by attaching an intravenous infusion, ensuring that it runs freely or using an injection of saline. The tissues around the site must be observed for any signs of swelling that may indicate that the cannula is incorrectly positioned. Finally the cannula should be secured in an appropriate manner.

CUTDOWN

Box 15.1   Equipment for cutdown

 1. Skin preparation solution
 2. Swabs
 3. Sterile sheets
 4. Sterile gowns for the nurse and doctor
 5. Local anaesthetic
 6. Syringe and needle for administering anaesthetic
 7. Scalpel and blade
 8. Suture and sterile scissors
 9. Small haemostats
10. Cannula
11. Giving set, attached to intravenous fluid for infusion
12. Dressing

1. The operator should identify the appropriate landmarks. In the case of the long saphenous vein, this is the medial malleolus; with the median cubital vein, it is the medial epicondyle of the humerus.
2. If time permits, use skin preparation and local anaesthesia. A 3 cm transverse incision is made 2 cm anterior or superior to the medial malleolus or 2–3 cm lateral to the medial epicondyle at the flexion crease of the elbow.
3. Using blunt dissection, 2–3 cm of vein is freed from neighbouring tissue. The distal end is tied off, with the suture kept in place to allow traction on the vein. Proximally a loop of suture is placed, but not tied, around the vein.
4. Using scissors or a scalpel, a small transverse hole is then made in the side of the vein and a wide-bore cannula from which the needle has been removed is inserted. The proximal loop is then tied around the cannula to secure it in place.
5. Placement in the vein is confirmed by either aspirating blood or the ability to flush without leakage or swelling of the tissues. The intravenous infusion is then connected and the skin closed with interrupted sutures. Finally a sterile dressing is placed over the operation site.

CENTRAL VENOUS CANNULATION

Whenever possible when performing central venous cannulation, the patient should be placed in a head-down position to dilate the vein and reduce the risk of air embolus. Many approaches and different types of equipment have been described to secure central venous access. This section describes two approaches (internal jugular and subclavian), using a single technique which can be used for either. The techniques described are successful in both experienced and inexperienced hands. No further justification of their choice is offered. For those already skilled at central venous cannulation using a different technique (with an acceptable rate of complications), carry on!

Seldinger technique

Although initially described for use with arterial cannulation, this technique is very suitable for central venous cannulation and is associated with an increased success rate. It relies on the insertion of a guidewire into the vein over which a suitable cannula is passed. As a relatively small needle is used to introduce the wire, damage to adjacent structures is reduced.

Box 15.2   Equipment for the Seldinger technique

1. Skin-cleaning swabs
2. Lignocaine 1% for local anaesthetic with 2 ml syringe and 23 g needle
3. Syringe and heparinized 0.9% saline
4. Seldinger cannulation set: syringe, needles, guidewire, cannula
5. Suture material
6. Prepared infusion set
7. Tape

Having decided which approach to use (see below), the skin must be prepared and towelled. Full aseptic precautions are necessary as a 'no-touch' technique is not possible.

1. The equipment to be used is then checked and prepared. In particular, the floppy end of the wire is identified and free passage of the guidewire through the needle is ascertained.
2. The needle is then attached to a syringe and percutaneous venepuncture made.
3. Once the vein is identified by aspiration of blood the syringe is removed, taking care to avoid the entry of air (usually by placing a thumb over the end of the needle).
4. The floppy end of the guidewire is then inserted into the needle and advanced 4–5 cm into the vein.
5. The needle is then removed over the wire, taking care not to remove the wire with the needle.
6. The catheter is then loaded onto the wire, ensuring that the proximal end of the wire protrudes from the catheter. Holding

the proximal end of the wire, the cannula and wire are inserted together into the vein. It is important never to let go of the wire.

7. The wire is then removed, holding the cannula in position.
8. A syringe may now be reattached and blood aspirated to confirm placement of the cannula in the vein.

If difficulty is encountered inserting the wire, the needle and wire must be removed together. Failure to do this may result in the tip of the wire being damaged as it is withdrawn past the needle point, thereby making withdrawal difficult. After 3 min gentle pressure to reduce bleeding, the needle can be reintroduced. Occasionally it may be necessary to make a small incision in the skin to facilitate passage of the cannula.

The subclavian vein – infraclavicular approach

1. The patient is placed supine, with arms at the side and head turned away from the side of the puncture. Occasionally it may be advantageous to place a small support (e.g. a 500 ml bag of fluid) under the scapula on the side of approach, to raise the clavicle above the shoulder.
2. Standing on the same side as that to be punctured (usually the right), the operator should identify the midclavicular point and the suprasternal notch.
3. Under sterile conditions the needle is inserted 1 cm below the midclavicular point and 1–2 ml of air is injected to expel any skin plug in the needle tip. The needle is then advanced posterior to the clavicle towards a finger in the suprasternal notch. The syringe and needle should be kept horizontal during advancement, aspirating at all times.
4. Entry into the vein is confirmed by blood entering the syringe. The cannula is then introduced via a guidewire as already described.
5. A chest radiograph should be taken as soon as possible to exclude a pneumothorax and confirm correct positioning of the cannula.

The internal jugular vein – paracarotid approach

This method is based on the fact that at the level of the thyroid cartilage the internal jugular vein runs parallel to the carotid artery in the carotid sheath and therefore rotation of the head, obesity and individual variations in anatomy have less effect on the location of the vein.

1. The patient is placed supine with the arms at the side and the head in a neutral position.
2. An attempt should be made to try to detect the carotid artery. Standing at the head of the patient, the thyroid cartilage is

identified and the fingers of the left hand used to palpate the carotid pulse. The right internal jugular is the one most commonly used initially.

3. Under sterile conditions, with the fingers of the left hand 'guarding' the carotid artery, a needle is inserted 0.5 cm lateral to the artery.
4. The needle is slowly advanced caudally, parallel to the sagittal plane at an angle of 45° to the skin, aspirating at all times.
5. Entry into the vein is confirmed by blood entering the syringe. The cannula is then introduced via a guidewire as already described.
6. If the vein is not entered at the first attempt, then subsequent punctures should be directed slightly more laterally (never doubling back towards the artery).

Although a chest radiograph should be taken it is less urgent than when using the subclavian vein, as the cannula is more likely to be correctly positioned and the incidence of pneumothorax is much lower with this approach.

INTRAOSSEOUS ROUTE

This route is indicated if other attempts at venous access in infants or young children fail, or if they will take longer than 2–3 min to carry out. It can also be achieved effectively in less time and with less skill than is required to carry out a venous cutdown.

Box 15.3   Equipment for intraosseous access

1. Alcohol swabs
2. 18 g needle at least 1.5 cm in length
3. 5 ml syringe
4. 50 ml syringe
5. Infusion fluid

1. Identify the infusion site. Fractured bones should be avoided, as should limbs with fractures proximal to the possible sites. The landmarks are: (a) tibial – anterior surface, 2–3 cm below the tibial tuberosity (Figure 15.5); (b) femoral – anterior surface, 3 cm above the lateral condyle.
2. Clean the skin over the chosen site.
3. Insert the needle at 90° to the skin.
4. Insert pressure until a give is felt as the needle penetrates the cortex.

227

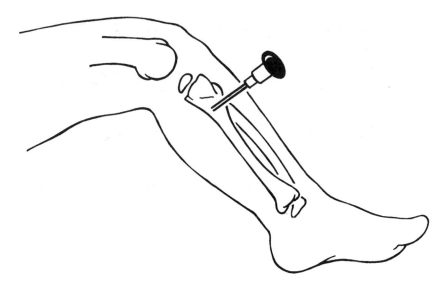

**Figure 15.5
Tibial site for
intraosseous
infusion**

5. Attach the 5 ml syringe and aspirate to confirm correct positioning.
6. Attach the filled 50 ml syringe via a three-way tap and push in the infusion fluid in boluses.

—16—
Practical procedures – treatment protocols

Procedures

- External pacing
- Defibrillation
- Cardioversion
- Needle thoracocentesis
- Chest drain insertion
- Pericardiocentesis
- Arterial blood sampling

EXTERNAL PACING

A pacemaker is a device which delivers an electrical current to the myocardium to stimulate depolarization and subsequent ventricular contraction. Internal pacemakers are the type most commonly used, but in an emergency external pacing can be performed.

Procedure

1. If the patient is conscious, they should be warned that the procedure may be unpleasant.
2. Self-adhesive electrodes are placed on the chest wall, anteriorly adjacent to the left sternal edge (similar to V3 chest lead for a 12-lead ECG), posteriorly beneath the left scapula and connected to the pulse generator.
3. The desired rate is selected and the output current increased until depolarization is stimulated.

The pulse generator is often a defibrillator which can be switched to pacing mode, or an additional module may be attached. Activation of the device usually results in considerable superficial muscle activity.

DEFIBRILLATION

Introduction

Defibrillation is the single most efficacious treatment of cardiac arrest in adults. In order to achieve the optimum outcome, defibrillation must be performed quickly and efficiently. This requires:

- Correct paddle selection
- Correct paddle placement
- Good paddle contact
- Correct energy selection

Many defibrillators are available. ALS providers should make sure they are familiar with those they may have to use.

Correct paddle selection

Most defibrillators are supplied with adult paddles (13 cm diameter, or equivalent area). For infants, 4.5 cm diameter paddles are used, and for children 8 cm diameter paddles.

Correct paddle placement

The usual placement is anterolateral. One paddle is put over the apex in the midaxillary line, and the other is just to the right of the sternum, immediately below the clavicle (Figure 16.1)

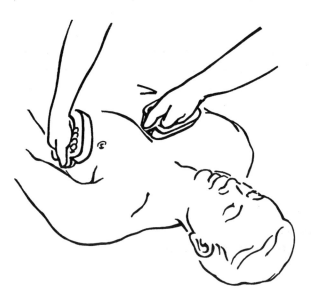

Figure 16.1 Standard anterior paddle placement

If the anterior-posterior placement is used, one paddle is placed just to the left side of the lower part of the sternum and the other just below the tip of the left scapula (Figure 16.2).

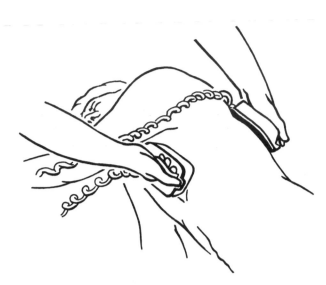

**Figure 16.2
Anteroposterior
paddle
placement**

Good paddle contact

Gel pads or electrode gel should always be used (if the latter is used, care should be taken not to join the two areas of application). Firm pressure should be applied to the paddles.

Correct energy selection

The recommended levels are shown in the relevant (adult and paediatric) VF protocols.

Safety

A defibrillator delivers enough current to **cause** cardiac arrest. The user must ensure that other rescuers are not in physical contact with the patient (or the trolley) at the moment the shock is delivered. Any GTN patches on the chest must also be removed as the energy delivered could cause them to ignite. If a temporary pacemaker is in use, ensure there is no contact between the external wires and the gel pads or electrode jelly.

Procedure

1. Apply gel pads or electrode gel.
2. Select the correct paddles.
3. Select the energy required.
4. Place the electrodes onto the gel pads or gel.
5. Shout 'Stand back!'
6. Press the charge button.
7. Wait until the defibrillator is charged then apply firm pressure to chest wall.
8. Check that all other rescuers are clear.
9. Recheck the monitor and deliver the shock.

10. Remember, discharge often requires synchronized pressing of buttons on each paddle.

When a permanent pacemaker is in place, the paddles must be placed at least 12.5 cm away from the generator box. Most modern permanent pacemakers have a built-in protection circuit to prevent damage during external defibrillation.

Basic life support should be interrupted for the shortest possible time (points 5–10).

Cardioversion

Preparation and performance of cardioversion are very similar to defibrillation described above. The main differences are:

1. If the patient is conscious, a general anaesthetic or appropriate degree of sedation will be required, administered preferably by a qualified anaesthetist.
2. The defibrillator is switched to 'synchronized' mode.
3. The correct energy level must be set, usually starting at 100 J.
4. The paddles must be applied firmly to the chest without movement to allow the ECG to be recorded.
5. When the buttons are pressed to deliver the shock, remember that there will be a slight delay to synchronize with the R wave.
6. Once the patient has been successfully cardioverted, the defibrillator must not be left in synchronized mode as this may inhibit its function if used for a patient in VF.

NEEDLE THORACOCENTESIS

Box 16.1   Equipment for needle thoracocentesis

1. Alcohol swabs
2. Large over-the-needle IV cannula (16 g minimum)
3. 20 ml syringe

Procedure

1. Identify the second intercostal space in the midclavicular line on the side of the pneumothorax (the **opposite** side to the direction of tracheal deviation).
2. Swab the chest wall with surgical prep or an alcohol swab.
3. Attach the syringe to the cannula.
4. Insert the cannula into the chest wall, just above the rib below, aspirating all the time.

5. If air is aspirated remove the needle, leaving the plastic cannula in place.
6. Tape the cannula in place and proceed to chest drain insertion (see later) as soon as possible.

If needle thoracocentesis is attempted, and the patient does not have a tension pneumothorax, the chance of causing a pneumothorax is 10–20%. Patients who have had this procedure must have a chest radiograph, and will require chest drainage if ventilated

CHEST DRAIN INSERTION

Box 16.2 Equipment for insertion of a chest drain

1. Skin prep and surgical drapes
2. Local anaesthetic
3. Scalpel
4. Scissors
5. Two large clamps
6. Chest drain without trocar
7. Sutures

Procedure

1. Decide on the insertion site (usually the fifth intercostal space anterior to the mid-axillary line) on the side with the pneumothorax.
2. Swab the chest wall with surgical prep or an alcohol swab.
3. Use local anaesthetic if necessary.
4. Make a 2–3 cm transverse skin incision along the line of the intercostal space, towards the superior edge of the sixth rib (thereby avoiding the neurovascular bundle).
5. Bluntly dissect through the subcutaneous tissues just over the top of the rib below, and puncture the parietal pleura with the tip of the clamp.
6. Put a gloved finger into the incision and clear the path into the pleura.
7. Advance the chest drain tube into the pleural space without the trocar.
8. Ensure the tube is in the pleural space by listening for air movement, and by looking for fogging of the tube during expiration.
9. Connect the chest drain tube to an underwater seal.
10. Suture the drain in place, and secure with tape.
11. Obtain a chest radiograph.

PERICARDIOCENTESIS

Box 16.3   Equipment for pericardiocentesis

1. ECG monitor
2. Skin prep and surgical drapes
3. Local anaesthetic
4. 20 ml syringe
5. 6 inch (15 cm) over-the-needle cannula (16 or 18 g)

Procedure

1. Closely monitor the ECG during the procedure. Look for an acute injury pattern (if not already present due to myocardial infarction) i.e. ST segment changes or widened QRS. These indicate ventricular damage by the needle.
2. Swab the xiphoid and subxiphoid areas with surgical prep or an alcohol swab.
3. Use local anaesthetic if necessary.
4. Assess the patient for any significant mediastinal shift if possible.
5. Attach the syringe to the needle.
6. Puncture the skin 1–2 cm inferior to the left side of the xiphoid junction at a 45° angle.
7. Advance the needle towards the tip of the left scapula, aspirating all the time.
8. Watch the ECG monitor for signs of myocardial injury.
9. Once fluid is withdrawn aspirate as much as possible (unless it is possible to withdraw limitless amounts of blood, in which case a ventricle has probably been entered).
10. If the procedure is successful, remove the needle, leaving the cannula in the pericardial sac. Secure in place and seal with a three-way tap. This allows later repeat aspirations should tamponade recur.

TAKING AN ARTERIAL BLOOD GAS SAMPLE

Precautions

It is important that these samples are taken and analysed correctly because their results can have major implications on the management of critically ill patients. Several iatrogenic errors need to be avoided.

Ensure an adequate sample

Samples taken from catheters must have the contents from their dead space removed first. A 4 ml discard is sufficient for samples taken from arterial lines and 10 ml from central venous lines or a pulmonary artery catheter. A sample volume of 2 ml is adequate.

Avoid excess heparin

The use of too much heparin can lead to marked changes in the blood gas analysis. It is adequate to fill the dead space of a 2 ml or 5 ml syringe, with the needle attached, with 1:1000 heparin. The use of preheparinized syringes is recommended.

Avoid contamination with room air

Remove froth and large bubbles and then seal the syringe with a cap. Allowing oxygen and carbon dioxide to diffuse in or out of the sample from a bubble can alter the level in the blood within minutes.

Minimize the effect of metabolism in the sample

Any delay in the sample will allow oxygen to be consumed and carbon dioxide to be generated in the syringe. If a delay to analysis of more than 10 min is expected, the sample should be stored on ice.

Obtain all available information

It is not possible to sensibly interpret the Pa_{O_2} in the sample until the inspired oxygen fraction (Fi_{O_2}) is known (see Chapter 4). Any recent bicarbonate therapy should also be noted. Extremes of temperature can affect interpretation of the results because the relationship between content and partial pressure will change as the sample's temperature changes. Consequently samples should be analysed at 37°C.

Avoid errors in analysis

It is important to use machines which have been calibrated daily and subjected to regular quality control.

Taking an arterial blood sample

As with any technique where there is the risk of blood contact, gloves must be worn.

Equipment for taking an arterial blood gas sample

1. Skin prep solution
2. 2 ml syringe, 25 g needle
3. 1% lignocaine
4. Heparinised 2 ml syringe, or prepacked equivalent
5. 23 g and 21 g needles
6. Syringe cap
7. Gauze swabs or cotton wool
8. Iced water

1. Identify the site of puncture, either radial, brachial or femoral artery. Clean and dry the area.
2. If the patient is conscious, infiltrate the skin and subcutaneous tissues with a small amount of lignocaine, taking care not to inject too much and obscure the artery.
3. Attach correct sized needle to heparinised syringe (23 g for radial or brachial, 21 g for femoral artery).
4. Confirm the position of the artery using fingers of your non-dominant hand.
5. Insert the needle, bevel upwards towards the artery at an angle of:

    30° to the horizontal for the radial and brachial artery
    70° to the horizontal for the femoral artery
6. Aspirate gently as the needle is advanced. This may not be necessary for prepacked, low resistence syringes.
7. Remove 1–2 ml of blood, then withdraw the needle swiftly and apply pressure to the site for up to 5 minutes.
8. Dispose of the needle safely and cap the syringe. Label the sample and send to the laboratory in ice water if there is any delay.

SECTION FIVE
Appendices

Appendix A
If you don't succeed

Objectives

After reading this chapter you should be able to:

- Identify the need for and the role of the relatives' nurse in the resuscitation team
- Achieve two-way communications with the patient's relatives/friends
- Understand the role of the police and coroner (procurator fiscal in Scotland)
- Deal with staff responses to death/dying and develop a philosophy of care for the suddenly bereaved

Ischaemic heart disease alone causes some 50/100 000 deaths per year in the UK. Many of those affected have no premonitory symptoms, and their first myocardial infarction is fatal. Death is therefore both sudden and unexpected. In such cases relatives and friends of the deceased are totally unprepared.

Failure to resuscitate also presents the medical and nursing staff with emotional burdens, at a time when they are clinically stretched and emotionally vulnerable.

EMOTIONAL CRISIS: NURSE INTERVENTION

Crisis is an unusual experience which most people will go through at some time in their life. It is an urgent and stressful situation which seems overwhelming at the time. However, with the right support from the beginning most people will come to terms with the experience.

The care of the relatives and friends of the critically ill or dying patient should be seen as important as the other tasks in the resuscitation team. The support for distressed relatives begins with their arrival in the ward or emergency department, and a trained member of the nursing resuscitation team must be allocated to this task before the patient arrives. This nurse must be able to concentrate specifically on the task once the relatives arrive.

During a crisis, family and friends often gather in the ward or emergency department. In the case of sudden death helpers are often just as devastated as the immediate next of kin. The relatives' nurse needs to be able to act and intervene, being informative as well as compassionate. The care relatives receive may well determine their mental well-being during the course of their grief.

The relatives' nurse should accompany the relatives and friends to a private room with suitable facilities available, i.e. telephone, tea-making equipment and toilets. Information useful to the resuscitation team may be gathered from them and this also gives the relatives the opportunity to express or explain how the patient collapsed. Likewise, the nurse can inform the relatives the severity of the patient's present state. By giving them time a rapport is begun, which will be maintained throughout their time on the ward or in the department.

Explanatory terms such as 'poorly' or 'critical' are meaningless unless accompanied by honest explanation. For example 'cardiac arrest' could be explained as 'His heart has stopped beating, he is not breathing and your husband may die'. This gives a better account than 'Your husband is very ill'. Of course, being with already distressed relatives and giving such information is not easy. This may explain why hospital staff tend to give limited information early on in any resuscitative situation. Nevertheless, if relatives are told exactly what is going on, they usually cope much better than if given a modified explanation or, worse still, no explanation at all.

It is an assumption on the part of many hospital staff that relatives may not cope with bad news. Experience has shown that given the facts, most people, though distressed, will deal successfully with the situation. It is when facts are vague that extreme reactions, such as anger and abuse, occur because the relatives feel excluded from the situation and no longer in control. A nurse assigned to the relatives in their crisis can build up a relationship of trust and be able to act as a link between them and the resuscitation team. This link is very important should the patient die.

The relatives' nurse should also allow a continuous appraisal of the patient's condition to be relayed to the relatives in a structured way. Honest answers to questions, with gentle explanations to what the resuscitation team is attempting, can be given. This nurse can also facilitate arrangements for the family, for example the distressed wife who remembers she has to collect the children from school, and be of further help when other relatives arrive.

SEEING IS BELIEVING

Should the relatives be allowed to see the patient? This is totally acceptable provided they are accompanied by the relatives' nurse and they are prepared for what they might see. Seeing with their own eyes helps them to come to terms with the event as it is happening. This may be the last time they will see their loved one alive, and so the encounter should not be prevented.

This type of policy can create personal issues for the team members. However, these views should not be forced onto others, what is right for one person may be completely wrong for another. Each set of relatives must be allowed to do it their own way while being guided and supported by the nurse.

THE PHILOSOPHY OF CARING FOR RELATIVES – CULTURAL AND RELIGIOUS ASPECTS

The ward or emergency department must have a philosophy for caring for the distressed relatives which is acceptable to their own locality with its various religious and cultural communities. There is no right or wrong way to proceed. Each family is different, but in each case their views and customs must always be respected.

COMMUNICATION – BREAKING BAD NEWS

There is no standard way of breaking bad news. However, if the relatives are treated with sensitivity and honesty from the very beginning it can lessen the impact when death has to be announced.

It is unfair always to expect the doctor to break the bad news. The nurse providing support is possibly in a better position to do this should the patient die because of the relationship that has been built up with the relatives. However, it is usual for the team leader to see the bereaved at some time. Before seeing the relatives the facts pertaining to the resuscitation should be gathered together, and some attempt made to remove any bloodstains or other marks that may increase distress. All the relatives' questions should be answered in as full a way as possible.

It is at the point of breaking the bad news that medical and nursing staff often feel inadequate. All that can be done is to listen and share the grief as it unfolds. There is no adequate expression which describes our feelings and concern – but sympathy must not be confused with sensitivity. Words spoken at the time of death will often remain with the relatives forever. Therefore choosing the correct words is important. When breaking the news, care should be taken to avoid using misleading statements. For example, '... I'm sorry we lost him' does not describe accurately that someone has died even though that is what is being communicated.

SAYING 'GOODBYE' – VIEWING THE DEAD PERSON

Following the death, the relatives must be given time to allow the information to be absorbed. Every conceivable emotional response is possible in any relative. The relatives' nurse must stay with them to guide them through the next stage of their stay in the ward or emergency department.

Shocked and numbed by the news, relatives may leave without saying their 'goodbyes'. Some will regret this in the future; therefore all relatives should be offered the opportunity to see their loved one.

They may never have seen a dead person before and consequently a great deal of fear may be present. The nurse can help displace these anxieties by active encouragement. It is important, especially when death has just occurred, to go with the relatives and let them touch and hold their loved one. If the deceased is a baby then a Moses basket should be available with suggestions given by the nurse as to the holding of their baby.

The relatives must be assured of plenty of time in order to say their 'goodbyes'. There can be no fixed rules and procedures; each family is different and the response must be geared to the particular situation. Their wishes must be respected and if a chaplain is required he or she should be notified.

If very invasive procedures have taken place, the team may wish to protect the relatives from viewing the body. Unfortunately, though well meant, these actions can lead to problems in the future. The family's fantasy of what the victim might look like could be far worse then the real thing. They have to come to terms with reality. Furthermore, a formal identification of the deceased often has to take place by law. It is better to explain the circumstances and let the relatives decide rather than impose your own perceptions on the family.

It is important that each ward or emergency department should be conversant with the local arrangements and have a good working relationship with the local coroner's officer. In cases of sudden trauma the deceased person will be deemed to 'belong' to the coroner until the cause of death has been established. This should not interfere with relatives saying their 'goodbyes' and holding and touching their loved ones. Where possible, the coroner's officer should be informed by the team leader and arrangements made for formal identification while the relatives are in the hospital. This will save them from having to return to the mortuary the following day and perhaps compounding their distress.

It is important for the nursing team leader to remember that the deceased's clothing should not be destroyed. This is not only from the point of view of the relatives, but also for legal reasons as the clothing may be required for forensic evidence.

THE ROLE OF THE CORONER

In most cases of sudden death, the coroner will make arrangements for the deceased to be removed for formal examination. Following this, he is obliged by law to hold an inquest if death cannot be attributable to natural causes. A post mortem may or may not precede an inquest, but if one is ordered by the coroner the person in possession of the body has no choice but to agree. The post mortem is usually carried out by an independent pathologist appointed by the coroner but interested parties have a right to be represented at this examination by a medical practitioner.

Inquests

These meetings allow the interested parties to ask questions of the witnesses called by the coroner. They are also open to the public and press. It is the coroner's officer who is responsible for preparing the evidence and organizing the inquest proceedings and, to this end, they must assemble all the statements and evidence.

Members of resuscitation teams are likely to be involved in an inquest at some stage of their careers. Evidence is usually given orally, with the coroner initially taking the witness through their statement, before they are cross-examined.

FURTHER SUPPORT

Ongoing support is needed for relatives. Written information may be required and should be readily available. The leaflet entitled *What to do After a Death* (Leaflet D.49) is useful.

The medical and nursing teams in the community should be

informed of the death and the clergy may need to be notified. A major asset in this follow-up care is a grief support nurse, who can act as a link between the hospital and the community it serves.

STAFF RESPONSE TO DEATH

Following sudden death in the ward or department, it is important to be able to acknowledge the distress among the staff. When actively involved in the resuscitation the team are often performing at their peak. Once the resuscitation has finished, especially if the outcome is death, then time must be taken to unwind. It is the practise in some wards or emergency departments to have an operational debrief to determine if the resuscitation team did everything that was required. It follows that an emotional debrief should take place, albeit informally, with the more experienced members being able to share their feelings with the less experienced. In this way no one person should feel ashamed of feeling sad or inadequate. It is far better to be able to share these feelings than 'bottling them up', as the latter can lead to days off duty from sickness or, ultimately, 'burn out'. It takes great courage to say one feels upset, and it takes a non-judgemental team who can share these feelings together so that they are ready to cope with the next critically ill person.

Developing a philosophy of care for the distressed relative and carrying out preventative emotional debriefing for all staff members reduces the future need for counselling, therapy and psychiatric intervention. Prevention is better than cure, and more cost-effective!

HELP GROUPS

All of these help groups have local contacts. The national offices will provide helpful leaflets and further information.

CRUSE – Bereavement care
126 Sheen Road
Richmond
Surrey
TW9 1UR
Tel. 0181 940 4818

The Compassionate Friends (An international organization of bereaved parents)
53 North Street
Bristol
BS3 1EN
Tel. 01272 539 639 (Helpline)
    01272 665 202 (Administration)

The Foundation for the Study of Infant Deaths
35 Belgrave Square
London
SW1X 8PS
Tel. 0171 235 0965

Stillbirth and neonatal death society (SANDS)
28 Portland Place
London
W1N 4DE
Tel. 0171 436 5881

The Samaritans (24 h support for the despairing)
Local branches in most towns in the UK.

SUMMARY

Sudden death is not an uncommon feature of resuscitation team work. Situations develop quickly over a short period of time. Relatives/friends are distraught and medical/nursing staff often feel inadequate. By addressing issues surrounding sudden death, developing a philosophy both as an individual and as a team member, will determine the care relatives receive at this time. Identifying the need for a special member of the team to liaise with the relatives/ friends – the relative nurse – makes communication easier for all concerned and subsequently the 'breaking of bad news' should become less erroneous. We have a duty of care to all, including relatives and friends, to allow them time with their loved one after death, give up-to-date information on legal requirements in sudden death, and offer adequate support locally.

REFERENCES AND FURTHER READING

1. Awooner-Renner S. I desperately need to see my son. *BMJ* 1991; **302:** 356.
2. Finlay I, Dallimore D. Your child is dead. *BMJ* 1991; **302:** 1524.
3. Lake A. *Living with Grief*. Heinemann, 1987.
4. McLauchlan C. Handling distressed relatives and breaking bad news. In: *ABC of Major Trauma* (ed. Skinner D, Driscoll P, Earlam R). *BMJ* 1990; **301:** 1145.
5. Werthaimer A. *A Special Scar*. Routledge, 1991.
6. Woodward S, Pope A, Robson W. Bereavement counselling after sudden infant death. *BMJ* 1985; **290:** 363.
7. Worden J. *Grief Counselling and Grief Therapy*. Tavistock, 1983.
8. Yates D, Ellison G, McGuiness S. Care of the suddenly bereaved. *BMJ* 1990; **301:** 29.
9. HMSO: What to do After a Death in England and Wales: A guide to what you must do and the help you can get. Benefits Agency,1995; HMSO, Norwich.

Appendix B
Ethical and legal considerations in resuscitation

Objectives

After reading this chapter you should be able to:

- Understand the legal background
- Understand the potential pitfalls in resuscitation

This article by Dr Patrick Dando was first published as 'Medico-Legal Problems Associated with Resuscitation' in the Journal of the Medical Defence Union, Volume 8, Numbers 1 and 2, 1992. It is reproduced here with kind permission of the Medical Defence Union and Dr Patrick Dando. All rights reserved.

The provision of resuscitation to a collapsed and perhaps unconscious patient is professionally demanding. As in any branch of medicine, the practitioner (any member of a resuscitation team) having taken on the duty of care to a patient is expected to provide a reasonable standard of treatment. Medical negligence may be alleged if there is a breach of that duty leading to a foreseeable injury to the patient for which the patient may claim compensation.

LEGAL BACKGROUND

Such an action is brought under the civil law of tort (meaning wrongdoing) under which a patient is compensated for injuries resulting from negligence. It is not appropriate to define absolute standards of care required from practitioners but, in the event of a claim of medical negligence, experts in the relevant field give opinions based on the circumstances of the case in the light of accepted standards at the time the events occurred. This follows the test of Mr Justice McNair who gave judgment in 1957 in the case of Bolam v Friern Hospital Management Committee and stated:

"The test is the standard of the ordinary skilled man exercising and professing to have that special skill. A man need not possess the highest expert skill at the risk of being found negligent. It is well-established law that it is sufficient if he exercises the ordinary skill of an ordinary man exercising that particular art."[1]

The jury were directed by Mr Justice McNair: "A doctor is not negligent, if he is acting in accordance with a practice accepted as proper by a responsible body of medical men skilled in that particular art, merely because there is a body of such opinion that takes a contrary view."[2]

A medical negligence action will not be successful if the injury results from the normal risks associated with that particular branch of care, nor is a practitioner expected to bring an exceptional level of skill but must apply the ordinary level possessed by practitioners working in the same specialty. It is understood that there may be more than one acceptable method of treatment.

It may be very difficult for the experts advising in a medical negligence action concerning resuscitation to distinguish between an injury caused by the illness which led to a patient's collapse and one which might have been caused by resuscitation. The experts called by the defendant and the plaintiff may hold different opinions. The issue may have to be settled at trial where a judge, on the balance of probabilities, will make a decision after considering the evidence.

During resuscitation, judgements may have to be made quickly concerning diagnosis and treatment. An error of judgement may not necessarily be negligent.

At the House of Lords in 1981, Lord Fraser, hearing the appeal in Whitehouse v Jordan, said: "Merely to describe something as an error of judgement tells us nothing about whether it is negligent or not. The true position is that an error of judgement may, or may not, be negligent; it depends on the nature of the error. If it is one that would not have been made by a reasonably competent professional man professing to have the standard and type of skill that the defendant held himself out as having, and acting with ordinary care, then it is negligent. If, on the other hand, it is an error that a man, acting with ordinary care, might have made, then it is not negligence."[3]

Training and supervised practice in the techniques and complexities of resuscitation are essential. Following proper instruction and supervised practice, self-audit is a great aid to improving technique. It is essential that a practitioner keeps up to date with new developments in resuscitation. Those responsible for supervising training must satisfy themselves of an individual's capacity to work in the field and ensure that any protocols are revised as new developments become part of standard procedures.

Earlier, in the Appeal Court, Donaldson L J had stated: "If a doctor fails to exercise the skill which he has or claims to have, he is in breach of his duty of care. He is negligent."[4]

Inexperience cannot be a defence to an action of medical negligence. Glidewell L J in Wilsher v Essex Area Health Authority 1987 said "... the inexperienced doctor called upon to exercise a specialist skill will, as part of that skill, seek the advice and help of his superiors when he does or may need it. If he does seek such help, he will often have satisfied the test, even though he may himself have made a mistake."[5]

This does imply that the inexperienced practitioner can recognize when help is needed. In an emergency specialist help may not be available immediately but should be sought when possible.

Practitioners who are not medically qualified must be particularly careful not to exceed the skills with which they have been accredited. Nor should they accept delegation of such responsibilities from their employers until they are satisfied in their own minds of their competence.

A person who unexpectedly comes across the scene of an accident has no absolute duty in British law to act positively for the benefit of others but most people would consider it an ethical duty, and the General Medical Council (GMC) states that the public is entitled to expect a registered medical practitioner to provide appropriate and prompt action upon evidence suggesting the existence of a condition requiring urgent medical intervention."[6] GPs as part of their terms of service are expected to provide emergency treatment to any person who requires it within their practice area.[7] A practitioner with special skills in resuscitation who offers assistance takes on a duty of care and must exercise it within the constraints imposed by the prevailing circumstances.

Since the introduction of NHS indemnity on 1 January 1990 doctors who work for a health authority are indemnified by their employer, which is vicariously liable for the acts of its employees and has to meet the costs for damages and legal expenses of a successful claim from its own budget. (GPs and doctors who treat patients privately make their own arrangements for professional indemnity through one of the medical defence organizations.) NHS indemnity does not cover health authority employees who provide voluntary professional assistance at accidents and disasters outside of their employment. Many doctors in the hospital and community services join a medical defence organization which can provide indemnity for 'Good Samaritan' acts as one of the benefits of membership.

POTENTIAL PITFALLS IN RESUSCITATION

A patient's condition may deteriorate rapidly, without warning and there is an obligation to identify any patient who is critically ill within an Emergency or other department and ensure that the patient is appropriately observed and resuscitation given with expedition if necessary.

A patient's collapse should be brought to the urgent attention of the resuscitation team who have to react immediately. The need for resuscitation may have occurred in the comparative luxury of a fully equipped and staffed resuscitation room or at a less convenient site, such as a hospital car park, a river bank or the patient's workplace or home. In these circumstances the resuscitation team must travel and take their equipment with them. Despite the urgency it is most important that the team does no harm to the patient, to others or to themselves. On arrival at the scene care is necessary to check for electrical, chemical and other hazards, which could have been responsible for the collapse and may present a danger to the rescuers. Appropriate action must be taken to eliminate such a danger.

With very limited exceptions a person suffering from an illness or an injury does not have to submit to examination or treatment if he refuses. However, if resuscitation is necessary the patient will usually be unconscious and unable to give consent. In an emergency the doctor should proceed and the treatment provided without specific consent must not be more extensive than that which is necessary to cope with the immediate emergency. If it is known that the patient would object to a treatment – an example would be a Jehovah's Witness who had clearly indicated the wish not to receive any blood product – that wish must be taken into consideration.

Clearing the airway from obstruction by secretions, vomit or foreign bodies, as well as its protection and maintenance is fundamental to resuscitation. While establishing an airway dentures should be removed and practitioners should take as much care as possible of the teeth during intubation. If a tooth is dislodged, it should be located and if it is not found this fact should be recorded and at a later date a chest X-ray can be taken to exclude the possibility of aspiration. The usual anaesthetic precautions should be taken to ensure that an endotracheal tube is appropriately sited and the possibility of oesophageal intubation is excluded. Oesophageal intubation is not necessarily negligent but on most occasions failure to detect it is. If there is inadequate respiratory effort, time should not be wasted trying a difficult intubation when other means of artificial ventilation are available.

Drugs and fluids may need to be given intravenously and care must be taken to ensure that the correct ampoule or bottle has been selected. A well-functioning intravenous line is invaluable and should be established as soon as possible. Certain agents, especially sodium bicarbonate, may act as an irritant if they extravasate and care should be taken to ensure that an intravenous line is functioning properly and has not been sited in an artery. It should be replaced if there are any doubts. When intravenous fluids are being given, care should be taken that they do not run through unnoticed.

Electrical defibrillation should be performed by somebody trained in its use and care must be taken that none of the resuscitators are in physical contact with the patient at the time of application of the electrodes. The patient's condition may warrant the insertion of a central venous pressure line, a hazard of which is that it may, albeit rarely, provoke a pneumothorax. This is not usually considered negligent, but the possibility should be borne in mind and excluded by a chest X-ray if necessary. The route selected by the doctor for the insertion of the CVP line should be that with which he is most familiar.

The unconscious patient cannot complain of pain and care must be taken that limbs are not placed in unsuitable positions with the risk of damage by pressure to peripheral blood supply or peripheral nerves or over-stretching of the brachial plexus. The head and particularly the eyes should be protected against inadvertent trauma.

In the course of resuscitation the practitioners will attempt to glean information, which is often limited, to establish a diagnosis and to provide appropriate treatment. On occasion the patient will carry a card or a 'medic alert' bracelet giving details of medication, allergies or of an illness, which can be extremely helpful. The patient may be carrying bottles of medication or a repeat prescription card from his GP which can be helpful and should be looked for, though it might need to be followed up in due course by a telephone call. Relatives or friends accompanying the patient can be a source of invaluable information and attempts should be made to identify and question them.

During resuscitation blood and other samples may be taken for urgent analysis and it is most important that containers and request forms are accurately labelled. If the patient's name is not known a reference number might be used. The specimens should be taken to the laboratory where staff should be informed that the results are required urgently. The requesting doctor is responsible for ensuring that the result is received and acted on appropriately.

It is vital to keep clear and concise records to provide detailed information to those who subsequently take on care of a patient. In the event of a medical negligence claim, such records will also provide proof of the facts of the case at some distant time. It is said that without a record there is no defence. The record should be made as soon as practicable and in some circumstances it is possible to designate one member of staff as the 'recorder' while resuscitation is continuing. It should contain relevant information on the observations made, drugs given with their dosage and timing, and details of the strength and timing of defibrillation. The record must be signed, dated, timed and be legible. It should be stored carefully together with any ECG tracing or pathology reports until they can be placed in the patient's file.

The patient who is successfully resuscitated will usually be transferred to an ITU and responsibility rests with the resuscitation team to pass on all relevant information. If possible this should be done orally and should be supplemented with a written record.

On other occasions the patient is not successfully resuscitated and close relatives will have to be informed. If a relative is near at hand, a private place must be found to explain what has happened. It is a difficult task which will usually be undertaken by a senior member of the team. If there is a request to see the body before it is moved, it may be possible to remove the various lines and tubes and make the body suitable to be seen; unless it is likely that the pathologist (or coroner) would wish them to remain *in situ* or has earlier made it clear that he would always wish for them to be left in place. The patient's property should be itemized and given to a near relative, who should be requested to sign a receipt, or it can be given a hospital administrator for safe keeping. On occasions the patient may not have been identified and assistance from the police may be required.

Sometimes it is possible for a medical practitioner to provide a death certificate if he has been in attendance during the patient's last illness. However, in every case of violent or unnatural death or sudden death, the cause of which is unknown, including a death following an accident, the doctor should notify the coroner immediately and will often be asked to provide a statement to the coroner's officer concerning the circumstances of the case.

On a few occasions a medical mishap may have caused a patient's collapse or one might have occurred during resuscitation. In that event it may be appropriate for the patient or the immediate relatives to be told of the facts by a senior medical member of the team. It is advisable to avoid speculation or comment on the actions of others. The simple courtesy of a sincere and honest apology may be necessary in certain circumstances.

The suddenness of a patient's collapse may be regarded as news-worthy by the public but the duty of confidentiality owed to a patient must be respected even after the patient's death. The media can be very insistent and sometimes it may be possible to answer queries by issuing a statement through the health authority's administration.

After resuscitation non-disposable equipment must be sterilized to prevent the risk of cross-infection. The usual precautions should be taken to avoid self-contamination by blood and other biological products. Used needles and other sharps should not be resheathed, risking self-inoculation, but placed into a sharps bin for later incin-eration. Hepatitis B immunization should be considered by any practitioner involved in resuscitation.

It is important that all equipment is checked regularly to ensure that it is functioning properly and that drugs have not become time-expired. The Consumer Protection Act 1987 requires a pro-ducer to ensure that a product is up to standard and fit for the intended purpose. If a patient suffers damage from a defect in a piece of equipment during the course of treatment, the liability rests with the producer who may escape that liability if it can be shown that the equipment was not maintained or calibrated or used in accordance with the instructions. The records for servicing must be kept for 11 years and are essential if liability is to be passed on to the producer in the event of the product being in some way faulty.

CONCLUSION

Through the competent application of their expertise the resuscitation team may draw upon the satisfaction of a job well done. If a patient dies, his relatives and friends will often appreciate that considerable efforts have been made in sometimes very adverse conditions.

REFERENCES:

1. [1957] 2 ALL ER 118 at 121.
2. [1957] 2 ALL ER 118.
3. [1981] 1 ALL ER 267 at 281.
4. [1980] 1 ALL ER 650 at 662.

5. [1986] 3 ALL ER 801 at 831.

6. Professional Conduct & Discipline: Fitness to Practise. GMC. February 1991: 10.

7. Terms of Service for Doctors in General Practice, February 1991, 4 (1) (h).

Index

Numbers in **bold** refer to figures and numbers in *italic* refer to tables.